ALLERGIES

**Questions
you
have
... Answers
you
need**

Other Books in This Series
From the People's Medical Society

Alzheimer's and Dementia: Questions You Have . . . Answers You Need

Arthritis: Questions You Have . . . Answers You Need

Asthma: Questions You Have . . . Answers You Need

Back Pain: Questions You Have . . . Answers You Need

Blood Pressure: Questions You Have . . . Answers You Need

Cholesterol and Triglycerides: Questions You Have . . . Answers You Need

Depression: Questions You Have . . . Answers You Need

Diabetes: Questions You Have . . . Answers You Need

Hearing Loss: Questions You Have . . . Answers You Need

Prostate: Questions You Have . . . Answers You Need

Stroke: Questions You Have . . . Answers You Need

Vitamins and Minerals: Questions You Have . . . Answers You Need

Your Eyes: Questions You Have . . . Answers You Need

Your Heart: Questions You Have . . . Answers You Need

ALLERGIES

Questions
you
have
...Answers
you
need

By Jennifer Hay

≡People's Medical Society®

Allentown, Pennsylvania

The People's Medical Society is a nonprofit consumer health organization dedicated to the principles of better, more responsive and less expensive medical care. Organized in 1983, the People's Medical Society puts previously unavailable medical information into the hands of consumers so that they can make informed decisions about their own health care.

Membership in the People's Medical Society is $20 a year and includes a subscription to the *People's Medical Society Newsletter.* For information, write to the People's Medical Society, 462 Walnut Street, Allentown, PA 18102, or call 610-770-1670.

This and other People's Medical Society publications are available for quantity purchase at discount. Contact the People's Medical Society for details.

Many of the designations used by manufacturers and sellers to distinguish their products are claimed as trademarks. Where those designations appear in this book and the People's Medical Society was aware of a trademark claim, the designations have been printed in initial capital letters (e.g., Claritin).

© 1997 by the People's Medical Society
Printed in the United States of America

Library of Congress Cataloging-in-Publication Data
Hay, Jennifer, 1964–
    Allergies : questions you have, answers you need /
  by Jennifer Hay.
       p. cm.
    Includes bibliographical references and index.
    ISBN 1-882606-71-X
    1. Allergy—Popular works. 2. Allergy—Miscellanea. I. Title.
RC585.H34 1997
616.97—dc21   96-29512
                                              CIP

2 3 4 5 6 7 8 9 0
First printing, March 1997

CONTENTS

INTRODUCTION

There's good news and bad news about allergies. The bad news is that they're easy to come by. Unless you've had a reaction in the past, chances are that you are unaware of the many things that can cause you to have an allergic reaction in the future. It might be a food that causes you to break out in hives. Maybe it's a neighbor's cat that makes your eyes water and your sinuses fill. It could be a plant you rub while taking a hike along an idyllic trail that, hours later, causes a rash up and down your arm. Allergens are everywhere. And as we become more sophisticated in terms of technology, we are always creating new products and chemicals to which many of us may be allergic.

But the good news is that most allergies are treatable. And with the right strategies, many of our allergic reactions are preventable.

And that is precisely why we published this book. *Allergies: Questions You Have ... Answers You Need* is your one-stop guide to understanding and taking charge of your allergies. Not only does it explain exactly what allergies are, how they occur and the best treatments for them, but it also shows you ways to lessen your chances of having allergies take charge of you. From the latest research to the most time-tested remedies, it's all here in these pages.

As the nation's largest consumer health advocacy organization, we receive thousands of letters every year asking for information. And since our founding in 1983, very few topics have generated as many questions as allergies. We have written about allergies in our newsletter and as part of many of our books, but this is our first book devoted exclusively to allergies. Why now?

The reason is simple. After looking at all the books and literature on the subject, we felt that an easy-to-read, easy-to-understand consumer guide was needed to help consumers make decisions about their allergies. As you'll note when you read the book, we are not promoting one form of treatment over another. The information found in these pages is directly from the medical literature—studies that show what works and what does not. The book is in question-and-answer format because consumers have told us they so often have not been given answers to their questions and often are not even sure of the questions to ask.

I am sure you will find that author Jennifer Hay has provided you with the most complete and useful allergy guide you have yet to use. We are convinced that with *Allergies: Questions You Have ... Answers You Need,* your ability to cope with allergies will only be enhanced.

Charles B. Inlander
President
People's Medical Society

1 ALLERGY BASICS

Q: What is **allergy?**

A: Allergy is an abnormal reaction to a substance that is usually considered harmless. These substances, which can be inhaled, ingested or even absorbed through the skin, are known as **allergens**. Hundreds, perhaps thousands, of ordinary substances can function as allergens. Among the most common are:

- **pollens**, the male reproductive cells of flowering plants, including trees, grasses and weeds
- **molds**, small fungi that reproduce by producing airborne **spores**
- animal **dander**, minute bits of sloughed-off skin
- dust, which can contain pollen, mold spores, animal dander, fiber and other allergens
- foods such as milk, wheat, eggs, peanuts, soybeans and shellfish
- medicines such as penicillin, penicillin-related antibiotics and **sulfa drugs**
- insect venom and secretions, including venom from stinging insects such as bees and substances secreted by biting insects such as mosquitoes and fleas

Q: Why does the body react abnormally to these substances?

A: It's essentially a case of mistaken identity. Allergy occurs when the body's **immune system**, which is designed to attack harmful foreign invaders such as bacteria, viruses and

11

parasites, mistakes a harmless substance for a harmful substance and attacks it in an effort to protect the body.

Q: What types of reactions does this attack produce?

A: Allergic reactions can manifest themselves in many ways and may involve any part or system of the body. When most people think of allergy, they think of the sneezing, runny nose, nasal congestion and itchy, watery eyes of what is called **hay fever**. But allergy can also affect the skin, the digestive system and the entire body. A person may react to an allergen by developing a rash, breaking out in **hives** or experiencing localized swelling. She may have stomach cramps or diarrhea. Or she may experience a dangerous systemic reaction known as **anaphylaxis**, which can ultimately result in shock and heart failure. And allergy often plays a role in triggering **asthma**, a chronic lung disease that affects more than 15 million Americans and kills an estimated 5,000 of those people each year.

Q: So allergy can be serious?

A: Yes. While most allergic reactions are not dangerous, some can be deadly.

Several hundred Americans die of **anaphylactic shock** each year. This most severe allergic reaction can be triggered by allergens ranging from insect venom, food and drugs to common respiratory allergens such as pollen.

Q: But serious reactions aren't the norm in people with allergies, are they?

A: Fortunately, no. For the vast majority of people, allergy simply causes discomfort and inconvenience. But that's not to downplay the significance of allergy, which in 1990 (the latest year in which these statistics were studied) accounted for more than 9.3 percent of all missed workdays and cost society more than $1.8 billion in direct and indirect costs, including lost

wages and health care. We say "more than" because the figures take into account only the costs of hay fever, or **allergic rhinitis**, the most common form of allergic disease. They do not include the costs of other allergic diseases.

Allergy also has a profound effect on the quality of life of its sufferers. According to a 1993 survey of 800 people who have allergies, conducted by the Market Research Institute of Kansas City, Missouri, 41 percent believe their quality of life is adversely affected by their allergies. This adverse effect is reflected in lost workdays, canceled social activities and altered appearance.

Q: How common is allergy?

A: Approximately 50 million Americans—1 in 5—have allergies, according to the National Institute of Allergy and Infectious Diseases. Hay fever alone prompted 9.2 million visits to the doctor in 1994, the latest year for which information is available from the National Center for Health Statistics. Asthma generated 31.9 million visits; **contact dermatitis** and other allergic skin conditions, 6.5 million visits.

The number of prescriptions written or shots given for allergy relief that year was 9.9 million. And that figure doesn't include the millions of over-the-counter remedies people bought to treat their allergies.

Q: Who develops allergy?

A: Allergy is an equal opportunity disease: It can affect anyone, regardless of age, gender, race or socioeconomic factors. Children are more likely than adults to develop allergies, but a first attack can occur at any age.

Q: Do people ever grow out of allergies?

A: Some people do. Allergies can change with time. Symptoms can improve or become worse, allergies can

disappear, or new allergies can develop. Many infants and young children with **eczema**, an allergic skin disease, outgrow it as they age, for example. On the flip side, however, many children with eczema develop other allergies later in life.

Q: So I take it allergies can't be cured?

A: Not really. As we said, it is possible for a person to grow out of an allergy or experience a reduction in allergy symptoms, but there is no medical cure for allergy. Fortunately, however, a variety of treatments and preventive techniques can be used to lessen the severity of allergy symptoms and bring allergies under control. We discuss treatment and prevention in detail in chapters 8, 9 and 10.

Q: Getting back to those kids with eczema who later develop other allergies, are they simply more prone to allergy than other people?

A: Yes. Some people are considered **atopic**, meaning they have a tendency to develop allergic reactions.

Q: Where does this tendency come from?

A: It is inherited. Although allergies themselves are not inherited, the genetic predisposition to develop them is. If one or both of your parents have allergies, you are more likely to develop an allergic condition.

Q: How much more likely?

A: If one of your parents has allergies, your chance of developing an allergy—any allergy—is 20 to 50 percent. If both of your parents have allergies, your odds rise to 40 to

75 percent. And if neither of your parents has allergies, your chance of developing them drops to between 5 and 15 percent.

Q: If I still have a chance of contracting allergies even if neither of my parents has them, I take it heredity isn't the only factor?

A: No. Although heredity plays a major role in determining whether or not you will develop allergies, it is not the only factor. Environment also plays a role. You must be exposed to an allergen in order to develop an allergy. We discuss this process, known as **sensitization**, in the next chapter as we take an in-depth look at the immune system and the mechanics of allergy.

Q: I've heard people say that allergy is caused by nerves. Is there any truth to that?

A: Yes and no. Allergy is not caused by nerves. It is caused by exposure to an allergen. That said, it's important to note that psychological factors can contribute to allergy. Emotions such as anxiety, fear, anger and excitement can make a person more susceptible to allergy attacks or increase the severity of allergy symptoms, as can stress, infection and diminished resistance.

Q: Wow! Allergy is pretty complex, isn't it?

A: It is complex—too complex to explain completely in this brief overview. We explore the complex mechanisms of allergy, its different manifestations, its triggers and methods for bringing it under control in the following chapters. It's a lot of information, so let's get started.

2 THE IMMUNE SYSTEM AND THE MECHANICS OF ALLERGY

AN OVERVIEW OF THE IMMUNE SYSTEM

Q: You mentioned that allergy occurs when the immune system mistakes a harmless substance for a harmful one. What exactly is the immune system?

A: The immune system is an elaborate network of organs, glands, tissues and cells that work together to protect the body from disease organisms such as bacteria, viruses and parasites. It protects you against diseases that you've already encountered as well as those for which you've been immunized. It also helps you fight infection once your body has been invaded by a disease organism.

Essentially, the immune system acts as your body's security guard or border patrol. It gives the once-over to the thousands of items you ingest, inhale or come in contact with each day, determines which things are potentially harmful and takes those invaders to task.

Q: Takes them to task? What exactly do you mean?

A: Components of the immune system work together to either destroy these invading substances or neutralize them—render them harmless. We discuss this in more detail later in the chapter.

Q: Good. In the meantime, I need to know more about the immune system itself. What parts of the body play a role in the immune system?

A: The major components of the immune system include the bone marrow and **thymus**, which manufacture and process white blood cells; the tissues, vessels, organs and nodes of the **lymphatic system**, which filters and conveys a fluid known as **lymph** and produces various white blood cells; and the white blood cells themselves. These blood cells, or **leukocytes**, are present throughout the body in both blood and lymph and play an important role in recognizing and fending off foreign substances.

Q: What exactly do they do?

A: There are several different kinds of leukocytes, and each plays a different role in immune response. Let's look first at the **lymphocytes**, the "foremen" of the immune system team.

There are two types of lymphocytes: **B lymphocytes**, or **B cells**, and **T lymphocytes**, or **T cells**.

Q: What do B cells do?

A: B cells identify potentially harmful foreign substances, then work to neutralize them, or render them harmless.

Q: How exactly do they do that?

A: When a foreign substance enters the body, the B cells are activated. They recognize the substance as foreign, multiply, then differentiate into plasma cells and memory cells. The plasma cells produce proteins known as **antibodies**, which attach to the substance and neutralize it, much in the way an acid neutralizes a base in a chemistry lab experiment. Foreign substances that can cause the body to produce antibodies are known as **antigens**.

Antibodies are specific; they are effective against only those antigens that brought about their creation. It may take some time for the body to produce adequate amounts of a specific antibody, but once it has learned to manufacture a particular antibody, it can begin to produce it again quite rapidly. And once the B cells have encountered an antigen, those that are transformed into memory cells "remember" the antigen, so the next time it is encountered, it can be attacked immediately.

This entire B cell process, known as **humoral immunity** because it takes place in bodily fluids, is how people acquire immunity to certain illnesses and is the basis of immunization. When a person is immunized against a disease, a small amount of antigen is introduced into the body. The introduction of this antigen into the body activates the B cells, which ultimately results in the production of disease-specific antibodies that neutralize the antigen. Once the antigen has been disposed of, these antibodies circulate in the bodily fluids, protecting the body against future invasions by that particular disease-causing organism.

Q: And the T cells? What do they do?

A: T cells, which are processed in the thymus (hence their name), initiate, direct and terminate a type of immune response known as **cell-mediated immunity.** When T cells encounter an antigen, they divide rapidly and produce large numbers of new T cells, each with a specific function. Memory T cells recognize the invading antigen; helper T cells stimulate the production of antibodies; killer T cells destroy the antigen; and suppressor T cells suppress, or turn off, the helper and killer and T cells after the antigen has been destroyed.

In terms of their actual disease-fighting actions, T cells stimulate B cells to produce antibodies and to attack and kill invaders within specific cells. T cells also produce chemicals called **lymphokines**, which stimulate **phagocytes** to attack and kill invaders. Phagocytes are cells that engulf, or ingest, microorganisms, antigens and cell fragments.

Q: Let me get this straight: These chemicals—lymphokines you called them—actually trigger this attack?

A: Yes. A number of chemicals are crucial to the function of the immune system. These chemicals, which are released from cells when an antigen meets up with antibodies or T cells, mediate, or act on, other elements of the immune system, triggering the next phase of an elaborate chain reaction. Because these chemicals act as go-betweens in this chain reaction, they are known as **mediators**.

Q: You said that other white blood cells also play a role in the immune system. Do these cells also release mediators?

A: Yes. Several other white blood cells act by releasing mediators into tissue and the bloodstream. These specialized white blood cells include **neutrophils, eosinophils** and **basophils**. The first two can also function as phagocytes, which as you remember ingest—and thus destroy—invading substances.

Q: So the white blood cells attack and kill foreign substances directly, release mediators and produce antibodies. I'm pretty clear on the first two. Could you tell me more about antibodies?

A: Certainly. As we've said, antibodies are proteins produced by the B cells. These proteins are also known as **immunoglobulins**. Experts divide them into five classes based on their structure and biological activity: Immunoglobulin (abbreviated *Ig*) G, A, M, D and E. **IgG**, the most abundant immunoglobulin in the blood, has antibacterial and antiviral properties and neutralizes toxins. IgA, which is present in the mucous membranes, provides antimicrobial protection in the body's respiratory, urinary and gastrointestinal tracts. IgM is the first antibody produced by activated B cells during the immune response. And **IgE** is the antibody responsible for allergy. (Experts are not yet completely sure what role IgD plays in the immune response.)

These antibodies either circulate in the blood and bodily fluids or attach themselves to certain cells.

Q: OK, I think I'm familiar with the players on the immune system team. Could you give me a play-by-play description of how they work together?

A: Certainly. The immune response begins when a foreign invader enters the body. Chemical mediators attract phagocytes to the site of the invasion. The phagocytes attach themselves to the invader and begin to engulf and digest it. At the same time, the T cells are activated. These activated cells secrete lymphokines, multiply and activate the B cells. The B cells, in turn, turn into plasma and memory cells and begin to produce antibodies. The antibodies bind with the antigen, neutralizing it, and a number of mediators are released.

Q: Is there visible proof that such a battle is taking place within the body?

A: There may be. Mediators provoke an inflammatory response. The area where the foreign substance invaded the body becomes hot as blood flow to the area increases and begins to swell as blood vessels dilate and fluid leaks into bodily tissues. If the area is visible, you may well see the results of this inflammation. And if the swollen tissues press on nerves, you may feel pain.

Q: Is that the end of the process?

A: In many cases, yes. But if the invader is stubborn and has managed to survive the attack, the killer T cells will launch a final assault, attacking and destroying the cell or cells that have been invaded.

Q: **How long does this process last?**

A: That depends on both the nature of the invading substance and the health of the person involved. It could take hours, days, weeks or, in the case of chronic illnesses, months or years.

THE MECHANICS OF ALLERGY

Q: **I now know more than I ever wanted to know about the immune system. But what is its connection to allergy?**

A: Remember, allergy is an immune system disorder. It occurs when the immune system mistakes a harm*less* substance for a harm*ful* substance and initiates the immune response.

Q: **You mean something totally harmless triggers that whole complex process?**

A: Yes. If you think of the immune system components as the body's border patrol, you can think of allergy as an episode of friendly fire.

Q: **Does this friendly fire, or allergic reaction, happen the first time a person encounters an allergen such as pollen?**

A: No. On first contact with an allergen such as pollen, the immune system simply produces IgE antibodies to counter it. No reaction occurs. These pollen-specific IgE antibodies attach themselves to basophils, which circulate throughout the body, and to **mast cells**.

Q: Another specialized cell? What are mast cells?

A: Mast cells are tissue cells. They are found in every tissue throughout the body, but they are most heavily concentrated in the skin, the lining of the nose and lungs and the gastrointestinal tract—areas often affected by allergy. Each of these cells is capable of hosting thousands of IgE antibodies.

Q: What happens after the antibodies attach to these cells?

A: The antibodies simply stay there, ready to spring to the body's defense the next time it comes in contact with the allergen. When enough antibodies are present on these cells—when the person becomes sensitized to the allergen—subsequent contact with the allergen will trigger an allergic reaction.

Q: What actually happens during an allergic reaction?

A: The actual symptoms of an allergic reaction vary depending on the number of IgE antibodies in the body, where the mediators are released and other factors. But the mechanics are essentially the same.

When allergens enter the body, they bind with the specific IgE antibodies that have been created to counter them. These antibodies, you'll recall, are located on the basophils and mast cells. When the antibodies and allergens bind together, the basophils and mast cells release chemical mediators. These mediators, in turn, increase the number of white blood cells at the site, spark a chain reaction that stimulates the production and release of additional mediators, and generate an inflammatory response. It is the inflammation of body tissues, caused by the chemical mediators, that creates the symptoms of allergy.

Q: Could you tell me more about these chemical mediators? How exactly do they cause allergy symptoms?

A: Let's start with the most well-known mediator: **histamine**. This chemical, contained in mast cells and basophils, is released when allergens bind with IgE antibodies. (IgE antibodies, you'll recall, are located on mast cells and basophils.)

Histamine causes small blood vessels to widen and become more permeable, allowing more fluid to pass from the blood into the tissues. This helps other white blood cells reach the site, but it also results in localized swelling. Depending on the location of this reaction, histamine can trigger nasal congestion, hives, a runny nose, itching and watery eyes.

Histamine also works with other mediators—specifically, **prostaglandins** and **leukotrienes**—to cause the involuntary muscles, such as those in the lungs and digestive system, to contract. This can result in asthma attacks and gastrointestinal problems.

Q: Are any other mediators involved in allergic reactions?

A: Yes. While histamine, prostaglandins and leukotrienes are perhaps the best understood mediators, they are not the only ones. Other mediators include heparin, which increases blood flow to the site of the inflammation; platelet-activating factor, which alters blood pressure; and bradykinin, which increases the permeability of blood vessels, causes smooth muscles to contract, lowers blood pressure and stimulates nerve endings.

Q: That's a lot of chemicals doing a lot of things. No wonder allergy symptoms are so diverse! Does anything else happen during an allergic reaction?

A: Yes. As we just mentioned, the number of white blood cells at the site increases. Chemicals released from the mast cells and basophils attract neutrophils to the site. The neutrophils generate destructive enzymes and a chemical known as arachidonic acid. These chemicals, released to attack the allergen, add to the inflammation.

Chemicals released from the mast cells also spark the production of an increased number of eosinophils. The eosinophils release chemicals as well. In this case, the chemicals trigger the basophils to release histamine, which increases the amount of histamine in the blood.

Q: **Does all this happen at once?**

A: Yes and no. As we said, the meeting of allergen and antibody triggers the immediate release of mediators and sparks a chain reaction that stimulates the production and release of additional mediators. Mediators that already exist, such as histamine, are released right away. Other mediators are produced or activated later in the process. While the existing mediators begin their work immediately, it can take some time for all of the components of the allergic reaction to fall into place. In fact, in some people, the reaction is not completed for hours.

Q: **I guess it resembles this explanation! I didn't realize how complicated this process is. Could you sum it all up for me?**

A: We can try. The typical allergic reaction occurs when a person is exposed to an allergen. The allergen enters the body, where it binds with IgE antibodies. These antibodies are attached to mast cells and basophils. When the allergen and antibody bind, mast cells and basophils release histamine and other mediators, while other mediators attract white blood cells to the site. These cells in turn spark a chain reaction that results in the production and release of additional mediators. The release of all of these mediators generates an inflammatory response, which takes the form of any number of allergy symptoms.

Q: **Is that it?**

A: Yes and no. In many people, the reaction ends here. In others, however, a second reaction occurs 6 to

24 hours after they are exposed to an allergen.

This late-phase reaction is triggered by a protein called **histamine-releasing factor**, or **HRF**. This protein, identified by Johns Hopkins University researchers in 1995, is present in everyone but affects only half of all allergy sufferers—people who have a certain antibody that reacts with HRF. The reaction of this antibody with HRF appears to play a role in the severity of the allergic response and how long it will last.

Q: Is there any way to tell which people react to HRF?

A: Johns Hopkins researchers are working to develop a test for the HRF antibody, which would identify the people likely to experience late-phase reactions. But since there is as yet no way to prevent these late-phase reactions from occurring, there is little practical application for the test.

In addition, the Johns Hopkins researchers say, other as-yet-undiscovered proteins may play similar roles in the severity and duration of allergic reactions.

Q: Just what we need—more factors to complicate this process! This discussion was complex enough, but I think I'm ready to get into the nitty-gritty of allergies. Can we get started?

A: Not just yet. There's still one type of allergic mechanism we haven't discussed—one that involves the T cells.

Q: I forgot all about them. Where do they fit in?

A: T cells are the primary players in a type of allergic reaction known as **delayed hypersensitivity**. This type of reaction is triggered by the meeting of sensitized T cells and allergens, not by the meeting of IgE antibodies and allergens, and it follows the pattern of cell-mediated immunity.

When the T cells recognize the allergen, they migrate to it and secrete mediators—in this case, lymphokines. The lymphokines attract phagocytes to the site. The phagocytes, in turn, begin to engulf and ingest the allergen. This process, enhanced by various mediators, eventually results in inflammation. We say eventually, because the inflammation generally appears after contact with the allergen—not immediately, as it does when IgE antibodies are involved.

Q: **What kind of inflammation does this type of reaction produce?**

A: Generally a skin reaction, such as a rash. Poison ivy is the most well known example of delayed hypersensitivity. We discuss poison ivy and similar reactions in more detail in chapter 5.

Q: **So are you saying that these delayed hyper-sensitivity reactions aren't as common as the ones involving IgE?**

A: Yes. IgE is responsible for the vast majority of allergic conditions. And in recent years, researchers have come to a much better understanding of the methods by which it works.

It is only recently that experts in the field of allergy and **immunology** have identified many of the players in the immune system and discovered what roles they play in the immune and allergic responses. Researchers are still attempting to determine the roles played by various chemicals, to pinpoint the specific genes that predispose a person to allergy and to uncover additional factors that contribute to the immune and allergic responses. The progress they've made thus far has given them a much better understanding both of the immune system and of allergy itself. But it has also shown them that they are dealing with an extremely complex system and an extremely complex disorder.

Let's go on now to see how doctors determine if a person is suffering from some manifestation of this disorder.

3 DIAGNOSING ALLERGY

Q: Is it important to find out the cause of an allergic reaction?

A: It can be very important. Remember, an allergic reaction occurs only when the body comes in contact with an allergen. If you can identify the substances your body recognizes as allergens, you may be able to avoid them, thus avoiding future allergic reactions. If you break out in hives every time you eat shrimp, for example, eliminating shrimp from your diet will prevent future outbreaks. Likewise, if you start sneezing every time you encounter a cat or dog, avoiding these furry friends—or at least limiting your exposure to them—will help ward off future sneezing jags or reduce the severity of your symptoms. You won't be cured of the allergy, but you will no longer experience its symptoms.

Q: But what if you don't know the allergen is present? How can you avoid it?

A: Good question. There may indeed be instances in which you know you're allergic to something but are unaware of its presence. Let's say you're allergic to coconut. You may consciously avoid foods with visible coconut topping but accidentally bite into a cake that has coconut in its batter, triggering a reaction. It's hard, if not impossible, to avoid a substance if you don't know where that substance might be found. In these instances, **desensitization** may help.

Q: What is desensitization?

A: Desensitization is the opposite of sensitization. It is the process by which your body loses its sensitivity to a specific allergen, and it is the principle behind **allergy shots**, which we discuss in detail in chapter 10. Needless to say, however, you need to know what exactly is prompting your allergies if you intend to desensitize yourself against those allergens.

Q: I'm convinced. So how do I go about finding out what I'm allergic to?

A: That depends. Sometimes the cause is obvious. Take the examples we just discussed: If you break out in hives every time you eat shrimp, you can be pretty sure you're allergic to shrimp. And if you sneeze every time you encounter a cat or dog, you can assume you're allergic to animal dander. Some allergies aren't as easy to pinpoint, however. In these instances, you may have to do some serious sleuthing, with or without your doctor's assistance, to find out what is causing your symptoms.

Q: Can anything other than allergy cause allergy symptoms?

A: Yes. A number of diseases share some of the symptoms of allergy. Tumors in the nasal passages, structural problems such as a **cleft palate** or **deviated septum** and even the common cold can produce nasal symptoms that resemble allergy. The autoimmune disease systemic lupus erythematosus and several kidney conditions can produce hives. And irritable bowel syndrome, stress, food poisoning and food **intolerance** can produce cramping, diarrhea and other gastrointestinal symptoms of allergy.

Q: So I guess it can be pretty important to see a doctor. Which doctors can diagnose and treat allergy?

A: Your family doctor, whether an internist or a family practitioner, or your child's pediatrician can often be helpful in determining whether symptoms are caused by allergy or by some other condition. Some family doctors will also help you determine which allergens are causing your problems and offer treatment. But the majority will refer you to an **allergist**, a doctor who specializes in diagnosing and treating allergy. You can also seek the services of an allergist yourself.

Q: Could you tell me more about allergists? What kind of training do they have?

A: Allergists are internists or pediatricians who specialize in the field of allergy and immunology. Also referred to as allergist-immunologists, they are licensed physicians—M.D.'s or D.O.'s—who are certified in either internal medicine or pediatrics. This means that they completed at least three years of full-time, postgraduate training in either internal medicine or pediatrics and passed a written examination in that field. These specialists then spent an additional two years in supervised postgraduate specialty training (called a fellowship) in the field of allergy and immunology. After they completed this training and passed a written examination, they could be certified by the American Board of Allergy and Immunology.

Q: What do you mean by certified?

A: The purpose of certification, according to the American Board of Medical Specialties, is to "provide assurance to the public that a certified medical specialist has successfully completed an approved educational program and an evaluation . . . designed to assess the knowledge, experience and skills requisite to the provision of high-quality patient care in that specialty."

Essentially, passing the board certification exam means that a doctor has been deemed worthy by his peers of practicing in his specialty. A board-certified specialist is likely to be competent in his field.

MEDICAL HISTORY

Q: **What can I expect during my first visit to an allergist?**

A: The first time you visit an allergist, or even the first time you visit your family doctor about allergy symptoms, you will probably spend a lot of time answering questions. The doctor will need to know information about your medical history and your family history. (Remember, the tendency to develop allergies is inherited.) Your family doctor may already have this information, but even she will probably bombard you with more questions.

Q: **What types of questions?**

A: The doctor will ask questions that reveal details about your symptoms:

- What symptoms do you have?
- Have you had them long?
- How long do they last?
- Are they severe?
- Do they occur at certain times of the day, at certain times of the year or when you are in certain locations?
- Do they occur after you've eaten or after you've eaten specific foods?
- Have you taken any medications to relieve them, and if you have, have the medications worked?

She may also ask questions about your lifestyle, such as:

- Has your diet changed recently?
- Have there been any changes in the medications you are taking?
- Have there been any changes in your job?
- Has a new pet entered the family?
- Have you been spending a lot of time outdoors?
- Have you been under any stress?

You might want to record this information in a diary. It will help you gather your thoughts and perhaps reveal patterns that can give you and the doctor clues as to what may be triggering your symptoms.

PHYSICAL EXAMINATION

Q: What else will the doctor do?

A: She'll probably perform a physical examination. Most likely, she'll listen to your heart and lungs, check your blood pressure and examine your skin, throat, ears, eyes and nose. Again, her goal is to rule out any other illnesses that may be causing your symptoms. She will also look for evidence of the symptoms themselves and any signs that indicate the presence of allergy.

Q: Such as?

A: Obvious signs and symptoms such as:

- a rash
- hives
- red or watery eyes
- sneezing
- a runny nose
- puffiness and darkness below the eyes (often called an **allergic shiner**)
- a crease on the bridge of the nose caused by repeated pushing on the nose to relieve itching (a motion referred to as the **allergic salute**).

She'll also look for less obvious signs. She may, for example, use a viewing instrument called a **rhinoscope** to observe the lining, or **mucosa**, of your nose. The mucosa is normally smooth and pink. If it is puffy and pale or purplish, it may indicate allergy.

LABORATORY TESTS

Q: Will she run any tests?

A: She might. If the doctor is unsure whether your symptoms are caused by allergy or another condition, she may run a series of diagnostic tests, including blood counts, x-rays, **pulmonary function tests** and cultures, to help her narrow down the cause. She may, for example, take a sample of your nasal secretions to test for bacteria and viruses. Or she may test those secretions for the presence of eosinophils, white blood cells that are plentiful in the nasal secretions of people with allergy. Again, these tests can either rule out other causes of your symptoms or confirm that you do indeed have allergies.

Q: Back up a minute! How does she get those nasal secretions? It sounds like it could be painful.

A: It isn't pleasant. The doctor places a large cotton-tipped swab, somewhat similar to a giant Q-Tip, into your nostril. Although this procedure takes very little time, it can make your eyes water and cause some discomfort. Remember, however, that these laboratory tests are performed only when the doctor needs to determine whether your symptoms are caused by allergy or by something else. They are not necessarily routine.

Q: Understood. Let's say the doctor is pretty sure that my symptoms are caused by allergy. What happens next?

A: That depends on the nature and severity of your allergy. If the cause of your allergy is obvious without testing— say, you sneeze whenever you pet a cat—she may tell you what you are allergic to and discuss with you the various methods that you can use to treat your symptoms or bring your allergy under control (methods we discuss in detail in chapters 8, 9 and 10). If, however, she is unsure of what is causing your allergy, if she suspects that you are allergic to more than one substance or if the type of treatment you opt for requires positive confirmation that you are indeed allergic to a specific substance, she will probably suggest that you undergo allergy testing to determine which substance or substances cause you to react.

ALLERGY TESTS

Q: What does allergy testing entail? Will I have to go to the hospital?

A: There are two major types of allergy tests: skin tests and blood tests. Both of these tests can be performed in the doctor's office.

Skin Tests

Q: Could you tell me more about these tests, starting with the skin tests?

A: Certainly. There are four types of skin tests: the **scratch test**, the **prick test** (or **puncture test**), the **intradermal test** (or **intracutaneous test**) and the **patch test**. The first three of these tests are used to determine if extracts of suspected allergens applied to your skin produce allergic reactions.

Q: How do the tests differ?

A: As their names imply, the tests differ in the way the extracts are applied to your skin—usually the skin on your arm or your back. In the scratch test, the doctor or his assistant makes a series of short, superficial scratches on the skin, then rubs a different extract of a suspected allergen in each scratch. In the prick test, the doctor places small drops of different allergen extracts on the skin, then uses a small needle to prick the skin under the drops. And in the intradermal test, the doctor injects a solution containing the allergen extract directly into the skin.

Q: That last test sounds painful. Do these tests hurt?

A: They are not comfortable, but they generally don't cause any pain. With the scratch test, you may feel a slight scratching sensation. With the prick test, you may feel a slight prick. And with the intradermal test, you may feel a slight sting as the extract is injected into your skin. Although intradermal tests do involve injections, the injections penetrate the skin only superficially (hence their name, which means within the skin).

Q: What happens next?

A: The doctor waits to see if the allergen extract produces a reaction. If in 15 to 20 minutes a red, itchy welt, or **wheal**, develops, it means you have reacted positively to that substance.

Q: Does a positive reaction mean I'm allergic to that substance?

A: It might. A positive skin test reaction indicates the presence of antibodies. The test shows that your body has been exposed to a particular allergen and has been sensitized to it. It does not, however, prove that you are presently allergic to the substance or that you would have an allergic reaction if you were exposed to it. It simply indicates that you have the potential to react to the substance. And there are instances in which a person is allergic to a specific substance but a skin test does not produce a reaction.

Q: If skin tests don't always prove that a person is or isn't allergic to a substance, why are they used?

A: Because in many instances they are the most effective type of test for determining a person's allergies.

Q: In which instances are skin tests most effective?

A: Skin tests are generally considered to be the most effective for detecting allergies caused by inhaled substances, such as pollens and molds, and by certain foods. They are also used on occasion to diagnose allergies caused by drugs, chemicals and insect venom.

Q: Which of the skin tests is used most often?

A: The most commonly used skin test is the prick, or puncture, test.

According to practice parameters for allergy diagnostic testing issued in 1995 by the American College of Allergy, Asthma and Immunology (ACAAI) and the American Academy of Allergy, Asthma and Immunology (AAAAI), the prick test is generally considered to be the most convenient, least expensive and most specific method for detecting the presence of immunoglobulin E antibodies in people with histories of exposure to inhaled and food allergens. The intradermal test is more sensitive than the prick test and is generally used when the results of a prick test are negative despite indications from a person's history or exposure that he is allergic to a specific substance. It is also used in infants and in older patients, since their skin is less likely to react to a prick test than the skin of children and younger adults. The scratch test, the original allergy skin test, is rarely used nowadays because it is the least sensitive.

Q: You said the intradermal test may be used if a person tests negative to a suspected allergen during a prick test. How many times does a person undergo skin testing, and how many allergens does a doctor test for?

A: The number of times a person undergoes skin testing and the number of allergens for which he is tested depend on several factors, including his history, the various allergens to which he may be exposed and the results of previous skin tests. Remember, prior to allergy testing, the doctor and patient have discussed the patient's medical history, including his allergy symptoms and the various allergens to which he may be exposed. The doctor uses this information to whittle down the number of potential allergens for which the patient will be tested. Patients who have histories that imply that they are allergic to more than one substance or who are exposed to more than the usual number of allergens will probably undergo more tests than patients who have less elaborate histories or who are exposed to fewer allergens.

The results of previous allergy tests may also play a part. As we've said, a patient who has negative skin test reactions to substances that his history or exposure implies he's allergic to may undergo additional testing.

Q: **You're basically saying there is no set number of allergens or testing sessions. Can testing go on forever, or is there some sort of upper limit?**

A: According to the ACAAI-AAAAI guidelines, evaluation for allergies caused by inhaled substances should require no more than 70 prick tests and no more than 40 intradermal tests. The number of skin tests performed for suspected food allergies can range from fewer than 20 to as many as 80.

Q: **How many substances is a person tested for at one time?**

A: Again, that depends on the specific situation and the site on the body at which the tests are administered. Up to 35 prick tests can be administered during one session. But the guidelines recommend that the number of intradermal tests performed in a single session be limited to avoid possible problems caused by multiple allergic skin reactions in highly sensitive patients.

Q: Are you saying these tests pose some danger?

A: Allergy skin testing is generally a very safe procedure, but it's not without risks. The most serious risk is that a person will experience an extreme allergic, or anaphylactic, reaction. Anaphylaxis, as you'll recall, is the most serious type of allergic reaction. It can include swelling, itching, difficulty breathing and a serious drop in blood pressure and can result in heart failure, shock and even death. Anaphylactic reactions are more common with intradermal tests than with prick tests. Fortunately, however, anaphylactic reactions to skin testing are exceedingly rare.

More common is the possibility that a person will experience a reaction at the site of the test that is more extreme than the expected wheal. The area can become swollen, red and itchy, causing discomfort. Doctors can reduce the likelihood of adverse reactions to skin tests by administering prick tests before intradermal tests, by diluting the allergen extracts they use and by limiting the number of tests they perform in a single session.

Q: Didn't you say there's another type of skin test—the patch test? Could you tell me something about it?

A: The patch test is used to diagnose **allergic contact dermatitis**, a skin rash caused by contact with an allergen. Poison ivy is the most well known example of allergic contact dermatitis; we discuss poison ivy in more detail in chapter 5. Other common allergens are nickel (used in jewelry), latex and a variety of chemicals that people come in contact with during the course of their work.

In allergic contact dermatitis, the reaction occurs some time after contact with the allergen, a situation doctors call delayed hypersensitivity. Because the reaction takes a while to occur, doctors cannot use the standard skin tests to determine the cause of allergic contact dermatitis. Instead, they affix patches containing the suspected allergen to a person's skin—usually the skin of the upper back—and leave them there for an extended period of time, usually about 48 hours. After that time, the person returns to the doctor, who removes the patches and examines the skin to see if any reaction has occurred. If inflammation or a rash has developed at the test site, the test is considered positive for that allergen.

As with other types of skin testing, a positive patch test reaction to an allergen does not necessarily indicate that that allergen is the cause of a person's symptoms. But a positive reaction to a subsequent patch test for the same allergen can help confirm the results.

Q: **Is there anything else I should know about these skin tests?**

A: Yes. The accuracy of skin tests can be affected by certain drugs. **Antihistamines**, for example, may prevent your skin from reacting to a substance to which you are allergic. Tricyclic antidepressants, ulcer drugs such as ranitidine (Zantac) and chronic high doses of **corticosteroids** (more than 20 milligrams a day) can also affect your skin's ability to react.

If you are taking any of these drugs, you need to tell your doctor before you undergo skin testing. He may direct you to stop taking the medication for a certain amount of time. Skin testing works best if antihistamines are discontinued between 24 hours and one week before the tests are administered; tricyclic antidepressants, between 7 and 14 days; ranitidine (Zantac), 24 hours; and chronic high doses of corticosteroids, between two and three weeks.

Q: **What if it's not possible for me to stop taking a medication?**

A: If you cannot discontinue taking a drug, your doctor may use blood tests rather than skin tests to diagnose your allergy.

Blood Tests

Q: What kinds of blood tests?

A: Doctors use several types of blood tests to diagnose allergy, most of which measure the amount of IgE in the blood. IgE, as you'll recall, is the class of antibodies that develop in response to allergens.

Q: How do these blood tests differ?

A: They differ primarily in the types of measurements they take and in the way the measurements are obtained. Some tests measure the total IgE concentration in the blood fluids, or serum. Others measure the amounts of specific IgE antibodies in the serum. The majority of these tests obtain these measurements by marking, or labeling, certain substances with radioactive isotopes, but other marking procedures can be used as well.

Q: That sounds complicated. I just need to know how these tests are used to diagnose allergy. Could you explain?

A: The first type of test—the one that measures the total IgE concentration in blood serum—can be used to determine whether a person has allergies. High levels of IgE in the serum can indicate the presence of allergies, although elevated IgE levels can also indicate other diseases, such as allergic bronchopulmonary aspergillosis, an inflammatory disease of the lungs caused by a fungus; human immunodeficiency virus, the virus that causes AIDS; and a form of bone-destroying tumor. The **radioimmunosorbent test**, or **RIST**, is an example of this type of test.

The second type of test—the one that measures the amounts of specific IgE antibodies in the blood—can be used to determine the substances to which a person is allergic. If a person has a specific IgE antibody in his blood, there is a good chance he may be allergic to the corresponding allergen. The **radioallergosorbent test**, or **RAST**, is an example of this type of test.

Q: Are these tests ever done together?

A: Yes. In fact, the ACAAI-AAAAI guidelines recommend that a total serum IgE test be performed on all serum tested for specific IgE levels to help the tester better interpret the results and to ensure accuracy.

Q: Which is better for diagnosing allergies— RAST or skin testing?

A: Although both can be used to diagnose allergies, skin testing is generally preferred.

Q: Why is that?

A: For one thing, RAST is more expensive than skin testing. For another, it is less sensitive. But RAST does have some advantages over skin testing.

Q: Such as?

A: Since the patient is not exposed to allergens during RAST, the test poses no risk of anaphylaxis. And since the test measures the amount of IgE in the blood rather than a bodily reaction, it can be administered to people who have been taking medications that might prevent the skin from reacting during skin testing. RAST can also be used in patients who have rashes, hives or eczema—skin conditions that could complicate, compromise or prohibit the use of skin testing.

Q: Are there any other types of blood tests that can be used to diagnose allergy?

A: Not exactly. There are several blood tests doctors can use to rule out other immunological problems that can mimic allergy, including tests that measure immunoglobulin G antibodies, serum immunoglobulin concentrations and other components of the immune system. There are also several tests doctors can use in conjunction with standard skin and blood tests to diagnose allergy in certain instances. These tests include **in vitro histamine release**, which detects the release of histamine from basophils in blood that has been exposed to an allergen in a test tube, and **in vitro lymphocyte proliferation**, which gives a picture of a person's cell-mediated immunity. At the present time, however, these tests are used primarily for research purposes.

Food Elimination and Challenge Tests

Q: Do doctors use any other kinds of tests to diagnose allergy?

A: Skin tests and blood tests are the tools most commonly used to diagnose or confirm allergy. But there are a number of other testing methods—some valid and some invalid. Some valid tests, such as **food elimination and challenge tests**, are simply used less frequently because they are limited to one type of allergy. But there are other, controversial testing methods being used today that are either ineffective or unproven.

Q: I guess I should know something about these controversial tests, but first could you explain the food elimination and challenge tests?

A: Certainly. Food elimination and challenge tests are used— often in conjunction with skin and blood tests—to diagnose food allergies. They can involve either removing suspect foods from the diet for a period of time, then reintroducing them one at a time and observing any reactions, or simply introducing a specific food to a person and observing his reaction.

Q: That sounds like something I could do myself. Is there any more to it?

A: That depends on the situation. If you suspect that a specific food is causing your allergy and your symptoms aren't life-threatening, there's no reason why you can't eliminate the food from your diet on your own, then reintroduce it and observe your body's reaction. But not all cases of food allergy can be handled this way. For one thing, some food allergies produce dangerous, anaphylactic reactions—reactions you don't want to trigger. For another, you may not really know whether your symptoms are caused by food allergy or by something else. Unless the situation is pretty cut-and-dried—you want to prove that shrimp cause you to break out in hives, for example—it's not a good idea to perform food elimination and challenge tests on your own.

Q: Understood. So how do doctors use these tests?

A: Again, that depends on the situation. If, after taking your medical history and examining you, the doctor suspects that you have a food allergy, she may suggest that you keep a **food diary** to help narrow down the possible suspects. In the diary, you would record all of the foods you eat, when you eat them and any symptoms that occur afterward. Once you come up with a suspect or suspects, the doctor might suggest a simple elimination-and-reintroduction food challenge like the one we discussed above, in which one food or perhaps several foods are eliminated and then reintroduced one at a time. The choice of foods to be tested is often based on the results of skin or blood tests.

If the cause of the allergy still remains elusive after these steps, the doctor might recommend a "blind" food challenge. In this test, which takes place in the doctor's office or even at a hospital under close observation, a suspected food or a neutral food, called a **placebo**, is given to you either in the form of a capsule or in a slush or pudding. This is done so that you don't know whether you are eating the suspect food or the placebo. You are, in a sense, blinded, so any psychological factors that may affect the results of the test are eliminated.

Q: **Psychological factors? Such as what?**

A: Such as your own personal belief that you are or aren't allergic to the food in question.

Q: **OK. What happens next?**

A: Your reactions are observed, and the process is later repeated with the food that was not eaten the first time. This type of test can also be performed in a double-blind fashion, in which neither you nor your doctor knows whether you are eating the suspected food or the placebo. This ensures that your doctor's preconceptions about your allergy do not affect the test results. Both the single-blind and double-blind food challenges are often quite helpful in establishing a cause-and-effect relationship between that food and allergy.

Other Allergy Tests

Q: **These sound like pretty definitive tests. What about the other tests you mentioned— the ones you said are controversial?**

A: The practice parameters for allergy diagnostic testing developed by the AAAAI and the ACAAI list the following tests as controversial: the **cytotoxic test, provocation-neutralization, electrodermal diagnosis, applied kinesi-ology**, the **reaginic pulse test** and **body chemical analysis**. Some of these tests are unproven, while others have been proven ineffective. Yet all are occasionally offered by some doctors.

Q: **Could you explain what each of these is and why it is controversial?**

A: Certainly. In the cytotoxic test, which is used to detect food allergy, the patient's blood is placed on a microscope slide that has been smeared with a dried food extract. The person performing the test then examines the blood cells under a microscope for any changes in shape or appearance. Changes supposedly indicate allergy to the food.

The ACAAI-AAAAI guidelines note that studies have shown the cytotoxic test to be ineffective. Both the Food and Drug Administration (FDA) and the Health Care Financing Administration—the agency that oversees the Medicare program—consider the test unproven. And in the December 1993 issue of *FDA Consumer,* the FDA warned that cytotoxic tests are often interpreted by "nutritional counselors" working on commission who then recommend the vitamins and minerals they sell to correct the patient's "allergic condition."

Q: **What about provocation-neutralization testing?**

A: Provocation-neutralization, which is used to diagnose allergy to foods, chemicals and inhaled substances, involves giving the patient varying concentrations of extracts of suspected allergens either by injection or sublingually (by placing it under the tongue). The patient records all subjective sensations for the next 10 minutes, and the person administering the test watches for any symptoms. Any symptom or reported sensation is considered a positive test for allergy. This is the provocation part of the test.

Q: **That sounds an awful lot like skin testing. What's the difference?**

A: There are several key differences. For starters, a provocation test can be considered positive if the patient experiences any subjective sensation. The development of an obvious sign of potential allergy, such as a wheal, is not required. In addition, the provocation test also includes a neutralization component.

Q: What does that entail?

A: If a positive result does appear after provocation, the person administering the test gives the patient another dose of the same substance in an attempt to neutralize the reaction and make the symptoms disappear.

Clinical studies evaluating this form of testing have found that responses to test substances are no different from responses to inactive, or placebo, substances, according to the ACAAI-AAAAI guidelines. In addition, the guidelines indicate that there is no rational explanation for this type of testing.

Q: Have the other tests the guidelines list as controversial also been proven ineffective?

A: No. In the case of the other tests, the controversy lies not with the results of scientific studies but rather with the lack of such studies. To date, no studies have been done on the effectiveness of electrodermal diagnosis, which measures changes in the electrical resistance of a person's skin when he is exposed to an allergen; on applied kinesiology, which measures changes in a patient's muscle strength before and after he is exposed to an allergen; on the reaginic pulse test, which measures a person's pulse before and after he ingests a food to which he is supposedly allergic; or on body chemical analysis, which measures various chemicals in body fluids and tissues. Further, the guidelines state, no rational basis or theory supports any of these testing mechanisms.

Q: Is there anything else I need to know about allergy testing?

A: Not really. At this point, it's time you learned more about the different ways in which allergy manifests itself. We discuss the major kinds of allergy—respiratory allergies, skin allergies and food, drug and insect allergies—in detail in the next three chapters.

4 RESPIRATORY ALLERGIES

Q: Respiratory allergies? That's hay fever, right?

A: In part. Respiratory allergies are allergies that affect the respiratory system—the nose, nasal cavity, sinuses, trachea and lungs, areas that are full of histamine-containing mast cells. This includes hay fever and other types of allergic rhinitis. It also includes asthma.

ALLERGIC RHINITIS

Q: That term sounds familiar. What exactly is allergic rhinitis?

A: Allergic rhinitis is an allergy that manifests itself in nasal symptoms (the prefix *rhino* comes from the Greek word for nose, while the suffix *itis* means inflammation). Typical symptoms of allergic rhinitis—the most common allergic disease— include swelling of the nasal passages, **rhinorrhea** (runny nose), nasal congestion, **postnasal drip** and **pruritus**, or itching, in the nose, throat and eyes.

Q: The eyes aren't part of the respiratory tract, are they?

A: No, but they are located close enough to the nose that they can be affected by the same allergens that affect the nose. And the membrane that lines the eyes, called the **conjunctiva**, is extremely sensitive to allergens. Many people with allergic rhinitis also have **allergic conjunctivitis**, an allergic condition that may include inflammation of the conjunctiva, itching and tearing of the eyes and extreme sensitivity to light. And these **ocular**, or eye, symptoms are often lumped in with the symptoms attributed to hay fever. Technically, the combination of nasal and ocular symptoms is called **allergic rhinoconjunctivitis**.

Q: Didn't you say that hay fever is actually a type of allergic rhinitis?

A: Yes. What we commonly call hay fever is officially known as **seasonal allergic rhinitis**. It is one of three types of allergic rhinitis. The other two are **perennial allergic rhinitis** and **occupational allergic rhinitis**.

Q: I take from the names that the difference among the three has to do with the time or place in which the reaction occurs, right?

A: Right. Seasonal allergic rhinitis occurs only during specific seasons—generally periods of time in which pollens are abundant. It's often called hay fever when it occurs in the fall, the season in which hay, or grass, is cut; many people are allergic to grass and weed pollens. Likewise, when seasonal allergic rhinitis occurs in the spring, when roses bloom, it is occasionally called **rose fever**. But the primary culprit in rose fever is tree pollen, not rose pollen.

Perennial allergic rhinitis, on the other hand, is triggered by allergens that are present year-round. And occupational allergic rhinitis, which is caused by allergens a person is exposed to on the job, can occur seasonally or perennially.

Q: Do the symptoms of these types of allergic rhinitis differ?

A: Yes and no. All three forms of allergic rhinitis can generate any or all of the symptoms we discussed. But not every person will experience every symptom. Generally speaking, people with perennial allergic rhinitis tend to experience more nasal congestion and postnasal drip than people with seasonal allergic rhinitis. In fact, they may develop chronic nasal obstructions that prompt them to snore or to breathe with their mouths partially open. Mouth breathing produces a dry mouth—a dehydrated environment in which bacteria can thrive. People with perennial allergic rhinitis are also more likely to experience complications.

Q: What types of complications?

A: The complications of allergic rhinitis can include **sinusitis**, an infection or inflammation of the sinuses; **nasal polyps**, bits of overgrown mucous membrane that extend into the nasal cavity, where they cause nasal blockages of their own; asthma; and blockage of the **eustachian tubes**, which can lead to ear infections and hearing loss.

Allergic rhinitis may also contribute to **chronic obstructive pulmonary disease (COPD)**, a permanent narrowing of the lining of the lungs. In 1996, researchers at the Boston University School of Medicine reported the results of a study that found that aging men with allergic rhinitis lost more lung function than did aging men without allergic rhinitis.

Q: Can a person have more than one type of allergic rhinitis?

A: Yes. In fact, it is quite common. Remember, some people are more prone to allergy than others. These people may develop allergies to seasonal allergens such as pollens and molds as well as to year-round allergens such as dust and pet dander.

Q: No wonder allergic rhinitis is so common! You did say that allergic rhinitis is the most common form of allergic disease, didn't you?

A: Yes. In fact, according to the federal Department of Health and Human Services, allergic rhinitis is the single most common chronic disease experienced by human beings. It is also the most common nasal problem in the United States, affecting an estimated 5 to 22 percent of Americans, according to a review published in the March 1995 *American Family Physician.*

The majority of people with allergic rhinitis develop symptoms before age 30. The peak incidence is in childhood and adolescence, although the disease can occur at all ages.

Q: **What allergens most commonly cause allergic rhinitis?**

A: Although foods, drugs and insect venom have been known to cause allergic rhinitis, the usual culprits, not surprisingly, are **inhalant allergens**—allergens that enter the body through the nose. The most common cause of seasonal allergic rhinitis is pollen. Common causes of perennial allergic rhinitis include molds, dust and animal dander. Occupational allergic rhinitis can be caused by any number of things, including chemicals, latex and the allergens mentioned above.

Pollens

Q: **I'd like to know more about the major allergens, starting with pollen. I know we discussed it briefly in chapter 1, but I need a memory refresher. What exactly is pollen?**

A: A subject of interest to the birds and the bees (particularly the bees), pollen is the small male cell of a flowering plant. It is necessary for the fertilization of the plant.

Q: **When you say "flowering plants," do you mean things like daisies and roses?**

A: Yes—but we also mean things like trees, grasses and weeds. In fact, the pollens of these three types of plants are the major allergy culprits.

Q: I never thought of trees and grasses as flowering plants. Why are their pollens so allergenic?

A: Trees and grasses—and many weeds as well—produce very small, light pollens that are designed to be spread by the wind. These pollens are present in the air we breathe and can be easily inhaled. (You'll remember that allergic rhinitis is generally caused by inhalant allergens.) In contrast, brightly colored flowering plants such as roses, daisies and goldenrod have large, heavy pollens that are carried from plant to plant by insects such as bees. These pollens are too heavy to travel easily by wind.

Q: How small are the pollens that cause problems?

A: The average pollen particle is under 50 microns in size— less than the width of the average human hair. Depending on the plant species, each plant can produce hundreds, thousands or even millions of pollen grains, which can be spread for miles by the wind.

Q: When are these pollens out there?

A: That depends on the type of pollen you're referring to and on where you live. Each flowering plant has an established pollination period. This period, which varies from plant to plant and from geographic region to geographic region, is when the plant produces and disseminates pollen. It is also when the plant's pollen triggers an allergic reaction.

Q: Can you give me a general idea when these pollination periods occur?

A: Certainly. Trees are the first plants to pollinate. In the south, their pollinating season can begin as early as January; in the north, it can begin as late as April. Generally speaking, however, the tree pollen season runs from February or March to April or May. Grasses are the next to pollinate; their season generally runs from May through mid-July. Weeds pick up where grasses leave off, pollinating in late summer and early fall.

Q: It seems like there's a pretty steady stream of pollen production. What happens if I'm allergic to pollens from all three types of plants?

A: Then you may experience the symptoms of seasonal allergic rhinitis from early spring into fall. Some people do indeed have this extended allergy season, but many people who have allergies to all three types of plants have more severe symptoms during one season or another. They may be allergic to several types of trees, for example, but only one type of grass or weed. Or they may be allergic to a plant with a short pollination period.

Q: So the specific pollens a person is allergic to play pretty strong roles in when he experiences allergy symptoms?

A: Yes.

Q: Then can you tell me which pollens are most likely to cause seasonal allergic rhinitis, starting with the trees?

A: The trees whose pollens commonly cause hay fever include alder, ash, beech, birch, cedar, cypress, elm, hickory, juniper, maple, oak, poplar, sycamore and walnut.

Q: What about the grasses?

A: Allergy-causing grasses include Bermuda, bluegrass, fescue, johnsongrass, orchard, redtop, sweet vernal, timothy and velvet as well as cereal grasses such as oats, barley and rice.

Q: And the weeds?

A: The primary culprit is **ragweed**, a weedy herb whose pollen is considered to be most responsible for late summer and fall hay fever in North America. Other allergy-causing weeds include burning bush, cocklebur, lamb's-quarter, mugwort, nettle, pigweed, plantain, Russian thistle, sagebrush and sheep sorrel.

Q: And each of these plants has its own pollination season?

A: Yes, although many may overlap. For more information on the various regional pollen seasons, see the chart on pages 54 and 55.

Q: You mentioned regional differences in pollen seasons. Are pollens more prevalent in some geographic areas than others?

A: There are regional differences, yes. Ragweed, for example, is more of a problem east of the Rocky Mountains. And the Southwest, once a haven for allergic Easterners, is now home to a number of allergenic grasses and trees.

Areas with cold, freezing winters traditionally have shorter pollen seasons, while areas with warm winters have longer seasons. The grass season in the south, for example, lasts all year. Perhaps the most pollen-free areas are those above 5,000 feet. Few flowering plants grow at this altitude, although pollen from lower areas can be carried in on the wind. The seashore is also relatively pollen-free; many airborne pollens blow out to the sea.

Q: Guess I'll be heading to the mountains or the seashore on my next vacation. But wouldn't a city also be a good destination? After all, there aren't as many plants in the city as there are in the country.

A: True—but cities are not necessarily pollen-free havens. There are grassy lawns in even the most urban areas, and many city streets are lined with trees. And as we said, pollens can travel for miles on wind currents. So while there may indeed be days when pollen levels in a city are low, there will also be days when the levels are high.

Q: Do the **pollen counts** I've seen in the newspaper include counts for each type of pollen?

A: Some do. Others provide information only about the total amount of pollen in the air. These counts are generally reported as the average number of pollen grains per cubic meter of air during a given period of time, usually 24 hours.

Q: Where do these counts come from, and what do they mean?

A: The counts are derived from collection devices—often coated glass rods—that are placed out in the air and rotated periodically. Pollens from the air stick to the surface of the rods, which are brought in after a period of time and stained to make the pollen grains visible. The grains are then counted, and calculations are made to determine the average number of pollen grains per cubic meter of air sampled and, occasionally, the average number of grains of each different pollen.

Pollen counts are used to determine when pollen seasons occur, so medical treatment for seasonal allergic rhinitis can begin at an appropriate time. Research has shown that people receive the most relief from allergy medication if they begin taking it before symptoms start. We discuss this in more detail in chapter 9.

Regional Pollen Seasons

Region	Allergen	Months
Arid Southwest . . . . southern Arizona, southeastern California, southern Nevada, southern New Mexico, southwestern Texas	Trees Grasses Weeds	February–June April–October February–October
California coast . . . . western California	Trees Grasses Weeds	January–June March–October May–October
Central plains . . . . western Colorado, southern Idaho, Kansas, western Montana, Nebraska, western New Mexico, North Dakota, western Oklahoma, South Dakota, northern Texas, western Wyoming	Trees Grasses Weeds	January–May April–July June–October
Eastern agricultural . . . . northern Alabama, Connecticut, western Georgia, southern Illinois, Kentucky, eastern Maine, western Maryland, Massachusetts, Michigan, western Minnesota, northern Mississippi, southern Missouri, eastern New Hampshire, northern New Jersey, New York, western North Carolina, Ohio, eastern Oklahoma, Pennsylvania, Rhode Island, western South Carolina, Tennessee, eastern Texas, southern Vermont, western Virginia, West Virginia, Wisconsin	Trees Grasses Weeds	February–June April–July May–October
Florida subtropical . . . . southern Florida	Trees Grasses Weeds	All year All year All year
Great Basin . . . . Nevada, western Utah	Trees Grasses Weeds	February–May March–October June–November
Northern forest . . . . northern Maine, northern Michigan, northern Minnesota, northern New Hampshire, northern Vermont	Trees Grasses Weeds	May–August June–August August–September
Northwest coast . . . . northwestern California, western Oregon, western Washington	Trees Grasses Weeds	February–June May–August May–September

Chart, continued

Region	Allergen	Months
Rocky Mountains	Trees	February–June
western Colorado, northern Idaho,	Grasses . . .	April–June
western Montana, mid-New Mexico,	Weeds . . .	May–October
eastern Oregon, eastern Washington,		
western Wyoming		
Southeast coast	Trees	January–June
southern Alabama, northern Florida,	Grasses . . .	March–October
southern Georgia, Louisiana, southern	Weeds . . .	May–October
Mississippi, eastern North Carolina,		
eastern South Carolina		

Adapted from: Peter B. Boggs, M.D., *Sneezing Your Head Off? How to Live With Your Allergic Nose;* Allan M. Weinstein, M.D., *Asthma: The Complete Guide to Self-Management of Asthma and Allergies for Patients and Their Families;* Stuart H. Young, M.D., Bruce S. Dobozin, M.D., Margaret Miner and the editors of Consumer Reports Books, *Allergies: The Complete Guide to Diagnosis, Treatment and Daily Management.*

Q: Can pollen counts tell you when the pollen is really bad?

A: Yes and no. Pollen counts as low as 20 grains per cubic meter may mean trouble for some people. Higher counts may mean trouble for still more people. But remember, most pollen counts reflect the pollen that was in the air during the previous 24 hours. Pollen counts can tell you whether pollen was bad the previous day, but they may not be able to tell you whether the pollen is bad at the current time.

Q: Do the counts really change that much from day to day?

A: Yes. The amount of pollen in the air can change rapidly. Variations in wind direction, humidity, temperature and precipitation can all affect the amount of pollen in the air. Thus, the most recent pollen count may or may not reflect the amount of pollen that is currently in the air.

Q: I understand how a change in wind direction could affect the amount of pollen in the air. But what effects do humidity, temperature and precipitation have?

A: Rain, particularly a gentle rain with small raindrops, tends to decrease the amount of pollen in the air. Temperature can either increase or decrease the count: Warm temperatures encourage pollination, while cold temperatures reduce pollen production. Likewise, high relative humidity weighs down pollen grains, making them less airborne, while low humidity lightens them, making them more airborne.

In other words, people allergic to pollen generally experience fewer symptoms on cool, calm, rainy days than they do on warm, windy, sunny days. Avoiding outdoor activities during the latter is one of several ways people with pollen allergies can control their symptoms. We discuss additional methods in chapters 8, 9 and 10.

Molds

Q: I'm sure such precautions are necessary with pollens, but what about molds? Couldn't I just avoid rotting things?

A: Molds do indeed grow on rotting things. But the fuzzy green coating that makes last week's casserole this week's garbage is not the only cause of allergic rhinitis. So keeping your distance from the refrigerator is unlikely to prevent you from sneezing. Mold is present in the air, both indoors and outdoors.

Q: How can mold be in the air?

A: Mold is a member of a group of plants known as fungi. These plants, which also include mushrooms and yeasts, reproduce by means of spores, microscopic particles that are distributed by air currents. These spores, which are common in both outdoor and indoor air, are the culprits of mold allergy.

Q: Do all mold spores cause allergic rhinitis?

A: No. Only a few of the many molds that grace our presence have been shown to cause allergic rhinitis. These include the indoor molds *Aspergillus, Penicillium, Mucor* and *Rhizopus* and the outdoor molds *Alternaria* and *Hormodendrum.* Unfortunately, this small clique gets around pretty well.

Q: Where are these molds found?

A: These and other molds are present in almost every possible habitat. Outdoors, they can be found in soil, vegetation, rotting wood, freshly cut grass, compost piles and piles of leaves, among other locations. Indoors, they are found in basements, bathrooms, refrigerators, wallpaper, humidifiers and air-conditioning systems, garbage containers, carpets, bedding, mattresses, pillows and upholstery.

Q: Are mold spores more prevalent at any particular time of the year?

A: Mold spores are not as seasonal as pollens: They are present in both indoor and outdoor air year-round, depending on geographic location. Outdoor molds can be found yearlong in the south and on the West Coast. In other parts of the country, they generally begin to appear after a spring thaw and hang around until the first frost. Generally speaking, however, mold spores are more prevalent—and **mold counts** are higher—in the warm summer months.

Q: Mold counts? Are they like pollen counts?

A: Exactly. Mold counts determine the number of mold spores per cubic meter of (outdoor) air.

Q: Are mold counts affected by weather the same way pollen counts are?

A: Mold counts are affected by weather, yes—but not always in the same way. Like pollens, some mold spores settle with rain and take to the air on dry, windy days. Others depend on rising humidity and rain to release them into the air. If you're allergic to outdoor molds, your doctor—or your own experience—can tell you the best and worst times for you to be outdoors.

Q: Is mold more of a problem in some areas than in others?

A: Outdoor molds are found in all areas of the United States. They are, however, more prevalent in agricultural areas and other areas where vegetation is plentiful.

Indoor molds are more common in moist areas, such as bathrooms and basements, and in older homes with damp rooms.

Animal Dander and Saliva

Q: You said animal dander is also a major cause of allergic rhinitis. Could you tell me again what dander is?

A: Dander is the sloughed-off flakes of skin from animals.

Q: Is dander an outdoor or an indoor allergen?

A: Animal dander may be present in the outside air, but it is primarily an indoor allergen. People who are highly sensitive to animal dander may react when they encounter an animal outdoors. But the strongest reactions generally occur indoors, in the animal's home—whether or not the animal is present.

Q: Why is that?

A: People who are allergic to cats or dogs aren't really allergic to the animals themselves—they are allergic to proteins in the animals' dander, saliva and, occasionally, urine. And these proteins, which are light and easily airborne, remain in the home even when the animal is elsewhere.

Q: I understand how dander and urine proteins can be present in the home. But how does saliva cause a problem?

A: Both cats and dogs groom themselves with their tongues, spreading saliva onto their fur. When they shed, they spread that saliva into the air. The dried saliva particles eventually make their way into the dust that moves through the air. They settle on exposed surfaces in a room but can be made airborne again by the slightest movement. Couple these particles with the dander particles the animals shed along with their fur, and you virtually fill a home with allergens.

Q: Which cause more problems—dogs or cats?

A: Cats beat dogs hands down. After all, they spend hours each day grooming themselves, spreading saliva with each lick. Members of more than 2 million American families are affected by cat allergies. But dog allergies also cause problems for families. After all, many people consider their pets to be members of the family, and few people want to constantly avoid their family members. A diagnosis of pet allergy can have more unwanted effects than the sneezing, sniffling, congestion and watery eyes of allergic rhinitis.

Q: I react only to my friend's cat, not to my own. Can a person be allergic to only certain cats or certain breeds of dogs?

A: No. If you're allergic to cat dander and saliva, you're allergic to cat dander and saliva—regardless of which cat produces it. Likewise, if you're allergic to dog dander and saliva, you're allergic to dog dander and saliva—regardless of the breed of dog that produces it. Some breeds of dogs do produce more allergens in their skin and saliva than others, while some breeds shed more dander than others. This increase in allergens can cause a person to experience stronger allergic symptoms when exposed to a certain breed of dog—but it does not mean that the person is allergic to only that breed of dog. If you're allergic to dogs, you're allergic to all dogs. And if you're allergic to cats, you're allergic to all cats.

Q: Then why don't I react to my cat?

A: Chances are you do react to your cat. Either you don't notice your symptoms or you don't attribute them to your cat. You may react more noticeably to your friend's cat because exposure to that cat increases your exposure to cat allergens and you then link your increased symptoms to contact with your friend's cat.

Q: Do any pets other than cats and dogs cause allergic rhinitis?

A: Although cats and dogs are the main culprits, people can develop allergies to gerbils, hamsters and rabbits. Horse-hair and cow hair, once used as stuffing in furniture, mattresses and padding, can also prompt allergic reactions, as can feathers—both those on birds and those in pillows and down stuffings.

Q: So what type of pet should an allergic individual have?

A: The safest pets for allergic individuals are animals that do not shed dander or have feathers, such as fish and turtles, lizards and other reptiles.

Dust

Q: Didn't you say that animal saliva particles can be present in dust? Are they responsible for dust allergy?

A: They can play a part. House dust is a mixture of many things, including allergens such as pollen, mold spores and animal dander and saliva. It also includes **dust mites** and their by-products.

Q: What are dust mites?

A: Dust mites are microscopic arachnids that feed on sloughed-off flakes of human skin (human dander, if you will). They live in carpets, mattresses, pillows, upholstered furniture and other household fabrics—anywhere that humans congregate.

Q: Do these mites bite?

A: No, but they encase their feces in an enzyme-rich coating that is highly allergenic. Dust mite feces, as well as their decomposed body parts, become part of airborne household dust and trigger allergic reactions in sensitized people.

Q: Are dust mites present year-round throughout the United States?

A: Dust mites thrive in temperatures of 65° to 70°F and humidity levels above 50 percent. Most parts of the country have temperature and moisture levels this high for at least a portion of the year. And unless homes are kept very dry, mites can thrive inside year-round. We discuss methods for ridding your home of dust mites in chapter 8.

Q: Do any other creatures contribute to house dust allergy?

A: Yes. In urban environments, the feces and decomposed body parts of cockroaches can pose problems similar to those posed by dust mites.

Other Allergens

Q: Do any other allergens cause allergic rhinitis?

A: A number of other inhalant allergens can cause allergic rhinitis. These include cottonseed and flaxseed, which may be found in fertilizers, animal feed, upholstery and some foods; pyrethrum, an insecticide derived from plants related to ragweed; kapok, a cottonlike fiber used to stuff mattresses, pillows, sleeping bags and life jackets; vegetable gums, which may be present in some denture adhesive powders, tooth powders, hair-setting preparations and cosmetics; and latex, which is a common cause of occupational allergic rhinitis.

Q: What occupations expose people to latex?

A: People who work in the rubber industry are exposed to latex, obviously. But the occupations with the greatest number of latex allergies are those in the health-care industry.

According to an article in the September 1, 1995, *Internal Medicine News,* approximately 7 percent of surgeons and 10 percent of operating room nurses are sensitive to latex. They are constantly exposed to the latex allergen, which attaches itself to the cornstarch powder inside surgical gloves. This powder, which is easily airborne, can trigger both allergic rhinitis and asthma.

Q: What are some other causes of occupational allergic rhinitis?

A: The causes of occupational allergic rhinitis depend, of course, on the occupation. Some are traditional allergens; others are limited to the workplace. Here's a rundown of some occupations subject to occupational allergic rhinitis and the allergens to which the workers are exposed:

- Animal workers (people who work in veterinary offices, in pet stores, on farms or with laboratory animals): Animal dander and urine
- Bakers, millers and grain workers: Allergenic proteins in flour and grains; molds
- Beauticians: Human hair and dander; airborne components of cosmetics; chemicals used to treat hair
- Food handlers and preparers: Plant proteins; dust from coffee and cocoa beans; vapors of foods to which one is allergic; molds
- Pharmaceutical workers: Dust and vapors from drugs to which one is allergic
- Printers: Chemical fumes and vegetable gums
- Textile workers: Cotton fibers; flax and hemp
- Woodworkers: Wood dust

Employees in many occupations are also exposed to a number of **irritants** that can trigger allergy-like symptoms or make allergy symptoms worse. These irritants, along with the allergens we've mentioned above, can also trigger asthma.

ASTHMA

Q: What is the relationship between asthma and allergy?

A: Asthma—a disease in which air passages in the lungs periodically become narrowed, obstructed or even blocked—can be triggered by allergy. Quite simply, the same allergens that cause hay fever can affect the lungs, causing inflammation, constricting the **bronchioles** and prompting **wheezing**. In fact, 40 percent of hay fever patients demonstrate some of these asthmatic changes during pulmonary function tests after vigorous exercise, even though they have no obvious asthma symptoms.

Q: Back up a minute. What exactly happens during an asthma attack?

A: During an asthma attack, the muscles that encircle the air passages in the lungs squeeze the passages, reducing airflow. These contractions are known as **bronchospasms**. At the same time, the cells along the airway walls produce a large amount of thick, gummy mucus, which can collect on the walls and narrow the airways. Finally, the lining of the airways themselves becomes inflamed and swollen, further restricting the amount of air that can pass through. As a result, when a person with asthma tries to exhale, he ends up wheezing or coughing to try to force air out of his blocked airways.

Q: And what sets this attack in motion?

A: An asthma attack usually occurs in response to a stimulus, or trigger—usually something a person has inhaled.

Q: Aha! So that's where allergy comes in, isn't it?

A: Yes. In a person with **allergic asthma**, or **extrinsic asthma**, allergens are what prompt an attack.

Q: How do they do that?

A: You'll recall that when an allergen enters the body and comes into contact with the immunoglobulin E antibodies, chemical mediators such as histamine are released, producing an allergic reaction. In a person with extrinsic asthma, the reaction displays itself in the form of asthma symptoms.

Q: Can a person experience both asthma and allergic rhinitis?

A: Yes. In fact, 30 percent of people with allergic rhinitis develop asthma. And allergy generally plays a role in most childhood asthma. More than 90 percent of asthmatic children under age 16 have allergies, as do 70 percent of asthmatic people ages 16 to 30. And in more than half of the cases of extrinsic asthma, there is a personal or family history of other allergies.

Q: Which allergens are known to trigger asthma?

A: Asthma can be triggered by most of the usual inhalant suspects—pollen, mold spores, animal dander, house dust, dust mites, cockroaches and latex—as well as by foods such as eggs, milk, wheat, corn, peanuts, soy and shellfish.

Asthma can also be triggered by viral infections, sinusitis, certain drugs, exercise and exposure to tobacco smoke, wood smoke, perfumes, household cleaners, household chemicals and other irritants.

Q: What's the difference between an irritant and an allergen?

A: In the case of asthma, irritants provoke an asthma attack by irritating the lungs and starting the cycle of bronchospasms, mucus production and airway inflammation, while allergens provoke an attack by stimulating the release of histamine and other mediators.

Q: How do infections, sinusitis, drugs and exercise trigger asthma?

A: For information about the nonallergic causes of asthma, we suggest you consult our book *Asthma: Questions You Have . . . Answers You Need.*

We address some of the measures allergic asthma patients can take to minimize their symptoms in chapters 8, 9 and 10. But first you need to know more about the other types of allergies.

5 SKIN ALLERGIES

Q: How does allergy affect the skin?

A: The skin is chock-full of mast cells—between 7,000 and 12,000 per cubic millimeter. Mast cells, as you'll recall from chapter 2, contain histamine and other mediators. If exposure to an allergen causes the mast cells in the skin to release these mediators, the resulting allergic reaction will affect the skin, causing it to break out in hives (known to the medicos as **urticaria**) or eczema (also known as **atopic dermatitis**). The mechanism differs in allergic contact dermatitis, as we'll explain shortly, but the equation is the same: Allergen plus skin equals rash.

Q: Does a person's skin have to actually come in contact with an allergen to produce an allergic reaction?

A: In the case of allergic contact dermatitis, yes. As its name implies, allergic contact dermatitis is a rash that develops as the result of contact with an allergen. But hives and eczema can be caused by allergens that are inhaled, ingested or injected as well as those that come in contact with the skin.

Q: Are allergic skin disorders common?

A: Yes. It is estimated that 20 percent of all people experience hives at some point in their lives. Up to 10 percent of infants and children and 1 percent of adults experience eczema. And countless individuals have experienced contact dermatitis courtesy of that famed three-leaved plant, poison ivy.

URTICARIA AND ANGIOEDEMA

Q: I'd like to know more about these disorders. Since hives are so common, let's start with them. What exactly is a hive?

A: A hive, or wheal, is a raised welt. These welts, which can range in size from between one and two millimeters to several centimeters in diameter, are generally pale at the center and are usually surrounded by an area of redness and warmth known as **erythema**. They are usually itchy, and they can last for up to 24 to 48 hours each, although they generally fade away in less than 24 hours. Sometimes they disappear without a trace, ending the episode; other times they are replaced by new hives.

Q: Where do hives appear?

A: Hives can appear on any area of the skin, but they are most common on the extremities and the face.

Q: What about that other term you used— **angioedema?** What is that?

A: Angioedema refers to large welts that appear below the surface of the skin.

Q: Do these welts look the same as hives?

A: Not exactly. Because the welt occurs deeper under the skin, you may not actually see it. You may see only the resulting swelling, which occurs most commonly around the eyes, lips, hands and feet and occasionally on the tongue and in the throat.

Q: The tongue and throat? Isn't that dangerous?

A: It can be. Swelling of the tongue and throat can block the airways and lead to asphyxiation. This is a medical emergency that requires immediate treatment.

Q: Does this happen often?

A: Fortunately, no. It occurs on occasion in people with both hives and angioedema. It can also occur during an anaphylactic reaction, as can angioedema of the respiratory tract. You'll recall, however, that anaphylaxis—a severe reaction characterized by hives, swelling, a drop in blood pressure, breathing difficulties and, on occasion, shock or cardiac arrest—is the least common type of allergic reaction.

Q: You said this swelling occurs in people with both hives and angioedema. Can a person have both at the same time?

A: Yes. In fact, they often go hand in hand. Approximately half of all people with hives have angioedema as well.

Q: Can we back up for a minute? You said that hives are caused by the release of histamine—the same substance that causes allergic nasal and respiratory symptoms. But the symptoms seem so different. How does histamine produce hives?

A: As we detailed in chapter 2, the release of histamine causes small blood vessels to widen and become more permeable. This allows fluid to pass from the blood into the surrounding tissues, which results in localized swelling. In the case of allergic rhinitis, the swelling occurs inside the nose, causing congestion. In the case of hives, it occurs in the skin, producing wheals. The dilated blood vessels are responsible for the characteristic redness and warmth of hives. And histamine's contact with the nerve endings in your skin is responsible for the itch.

Q: **You said that the wheals may disappear, only to be replaced by new ones. How long can this cycle last?**

A: A long time.
Hives can be either acute or chronic. An episode is considered acute if the cycle lasts for less than six weeks. It is considered chronic if the cycle lasts for more than six weeks.

Q: **Six weeks! A case of hives can last longer than six weeks?**

A: Yes. Although most cases of chronic hives resolve in less than a year, they can persist for a decade or longer and do so in approximately 10 percent of people who experience them.

Q: **Are these instances of chronic hives caused by long-term exposure to allergens?**

A: Possibly. In most instances, however, chronic hives are **idiopathic**, meaning they are of unknown origin.

Q: **Do you mean that the doctor can't identify the allergen that's causing hives or that she can't determine whether or not the hives are caused by allergy?**

A: We mean both. In some instances, the doctor may be able to determine that hives are indeed caused by allergy but unable to pinpoint the responsible allergen or allergens. In other instances, the doctor may not be able to determine whether the hives are caused by allergy or by some other condition.

Q: What conditions other than allergy cause hives?

A: Hives and angioedema can be caused by physical stimuli such as heat, cold and pressure; by systemic rheumatic diseases such as systemic lupus erythematosus and Sjögren's syndrome; by infectious diseases such as hepatitis B and mononucleosis; by the use of drugs that directly cause mast cells to release mediators; and by the use of drugs that affect the body's metabolism of arachidonic acid, a fatty acid that forms the building block of some prostaglandins. Angioedema without hives can also be inherited.

Allergic Causes

Q: No wonder it's difficult to nail down the cause! But why is it so difficult to pinpoint the responsible allergen when hives are caused by allergy?

A: Unlike respiratory allergies, which are generally caused by inhalant allergens, hives can be caused by allergens that are inhaled, ingested or injected. Many of these allergens can make their way throughout the entire body, causing a systemic allergic reaction. When an allergic reaction is systemic, it can be difficult to pinpoint how the allergen entered the body. And even if you are able to determine how the allergen entered the body, you may still have difficulty pinpointing the allergen itself. It could be something you ate—but is it something you ate today or something you ate yesterday? Is it something you were consciously aware of eating, such as shrimp, or something you were unaware of, such as a food additive?

Q: I think I understand. It's sort of like solving a mystery. But I don't have all of the clues yet. Are there any allergens in particular that commonly cause hives?

A: There are. The allergens that most commonly cause hives are foods, drugs and insect venom or deposits.

Q: **Could you tell me more about the foods that cause hives?**

A: Certainly. Food allergy is one of the most frequent causes of acute hives. The foods most commonly associated with hives include shellfish, peanuts, eggs, wheat, tomatoes, strawberries and milk. Hives can also be caused by food additives, preservatives and dyes as well as by antibiotics, enzymes and vegetable gums in foods.

Q: **How much of these items does a person have to eat in order to develop hives?**

A: The answer varies according to the severity of the allergy and the potency of the allergen. Some people have been known to react to peanuts, a potent allergen, simply by eating a food prepared in a dish that previously held peanuts.

Q: **What about drugs?**

A: A number of medications are known to cause hives. In fact, almost every medication can cause hives in one person or another. The prime culprits, however, are penicillin, sulfa antibiotics, **diuretics** and certain local anesthetics.

Q: **And insect venom?**

A: Stings from members of the insect family known as **Hymenoptera**—which includes honeybees, yellow jackets and fire ants—are a common cause of hives, as are the anticoagulants that mosquitoes and fleas deposit in the skin when they bite and the saliva of the kissing bug.

We discuss allergies to foods, drugs and insects in more detail in the next chapter.

Q: Do any other types of allergens cause hives?

A: Yes. As we mentioned, inhalant allergens and allergens with which one comes in physical contact can occasionally cause hives. People who are allergic to pollen tend to have more difficulty with hives during the pollen season. And animal dander and dust mites have been known to cause hives on occasion. Likewise, physical contact with grass or other allergens can produce hives.

Physical Causes

Q: Did you say that physical stimuli can also cause hives?

A: Yes. The so-called physical allergies—allergic-type reactions to physical stimuli—include **cold urticaria**, **cholinergic urticaria**, **exercise-induced anaphylaxis**, **pressure urticaria**, **dermatographism**, **solar urticaria** and **aquagenic urticaria**.

Q: Could you tell me a little about each of them, starting with cold urticaria?

A: Certainly. Cold urticaria, as its name implies, is caused by exposure to cold. The hives, which are usually red, itchy and swollen, develop within several minutes of exposure to cold—cold air, cold water or cold food or drink. Only areas exposed to the cold are affected, although a systemic reaction (anaphylaxis) can occur if the area exposed to the cold is very large—if the person swims in cold water, for instance. In general, however, these hives are harmless and short-lived, disappearing within one to two hours.

Q: What about cholinergic urticaria?

A: Cholinergic urticaria occurs when the body's core temperature is heated, either by direct exposure to heat or hot water or by exercise or anxiety. Cholinergic hives are generally very small, round and itchy. These hives are often brought on by a hot shower or bath and are often mistaken for an allergy to soap or shampoo.

Q: Is this the type of hives that provokes exercise-induced anaphylaxis?

A: No. Exercise-induced anaphylaxis, in which vigorous physical exertion produces hives and, later, respiratory and gastrointestinal symptoms (and occasionally vascular collapse), is not caused by an elevation of the core body temperature. And the hives it produces are generally large.

Q: Then what does cause this condition?

A: In nearly half of the people affected by exercise-induced anaphylaxis, symptoms develop only when exercise occurs within a few hours after they have ingested a food to which they test allergic. In other people, symptoms occur when they exercise after a meal, no matter what food they've eaten. And in still others, the reaction follows ingestion of aspirin or another **nonsteroidal anti-inflammatory drug (NSAID)**.

Q: What about pressure urticaria?

A: Pressure urticaria occurs in people whose skin is sensitive to pressure. The most common form of this is called dermatographism. In dermatographism, which affects up to 5 percent of the population, hives develop at the site of firm stroking on the skin. People with dermatographism can actually write or draw on their skin by stroking on it: The area on which they have "written" becomes red, swollen and itchy.

In other instances, pressure urticaria develops anywhere the skin is under pressure—under tight clothing or elastic, for example.

Q: **What about solar urticaria? Is it caused by the sun?**

A: It can be. In solar urticaria, exposure to certain forms of light, including sunlight, causes hives to appear. Artificial light can also provoke this reaction, which, fortunately, is rare.

Q: **And aquagenic urticaria?**

A: Aquagenic urticaria, another rare condition, is triggered by immersion in water, regardless of its temperature.

Q: **There certainly are a lot of possible causes of hives. But didn't you say the cause often remains unknown?**

A: Yes. While the cause of acute hives is often easy to pinpoint, the cause of chronic hives often remains unknown. In fact, according to a review of allergic skin disorders, published in the November 25, 1992, *Journal of the American Medical Association,* the cause of chronic hives is found in less than 5 to 10 percent of patients.

Fortunately, however, medical treatment for hives is similar regardless of the cause, as we will see in chapter 9.

ATOPIC DERMATITIS

Q: Atopic dermatitis—that's eczema, right?

A: Right. Atopic dermatitis is a rash that appears in atopic individuals—individuals with an inherited tendency to develop allergies—and is often associated with a specific allergy. It is often called eczema, from the Greek for "to boil over" or "to erupt." The word refers to the inflammation and weeping of the rash, which can be very itchy.

Q: Is this rash similar to hives?

A: It is similar in that there is redness, warmth, swelling and itching, but it generally does not include actual wheals. In addition, the rash can persist for long periods of time. When it does, it causes the skin to become scaly, thick and hard, a process known as **lichenification**.

Q: Where does this rash appear?

A: That depends on the age of the person affected. In infants, atopic dermatitis usually appears on the face, arms and legs; in older children and adults, it appears on the extremities, neck and upper trunk.

Q: Is eczema common in children?

A: Yes. More than 85 percent of patients with atopic dermatitis develop the condition in their first five years of life. And in fact, the course of the disease can be divided into phases based on age.

Q: What is the first phase?

A: The first phase is the infantile phase, which begins at four to six months. This phase is characterized by a rash on the face and, later, on the abdomen, forearms and legs. It may either resolve spontaneously or progress into the child-hood phase.

Q: Couldn't it be treated so that it doesn't progress into the next stage?

A: While eczema can be treated, treatment doesn't prevent it from progressing. It simply relieves the itch and helps clear up the skin during flare-ups of the rash. Eczema is a chronic condition, which may or may not persist through the various phases.

Q: Understood. What happens in the childhood phase?

A: In this phase, the rash is characterized by small, itchy bumps, dry skin and a thickening or hardening of the skin. It most commonly appears on the insides of the elbows, the backs of the knees and the backs of the hands and feet. The rash often improves during puberty, but it can persist into adulthood.

Q: What are the symptoms of adult eczema?

A: In adults, the rash is itchy, and the skin is thick and hard.

Q: What causes atopic dermatitis?

A: Researchers are still trying to discover the exact mech-anisms that cause atopic dermatitis. Studies indicate that the immune systems of people with atopic dermatitis are slightly abnormal. These people may have abnormal lymphocytes and mast cells in their skin. They may have abnormal blood flow to their skin. And their cellular immunity may be impaired, making them more susceptible to developing viral and bacterial skin infections. (Skin infections are a common complication of atopic dermatitis.) Despite these findings, however, the exact cause remains unknown.

Q: What about allergy?

A: Allergy appears to play a strong role in atopic dermatitis. The majority of people with atopic dermatitis—80 percent—have high levels of immunoglobulin E antibodies in their blood. Many show an unusual number of positive results when given skin tests for allergies. In some individuals, allergic sensitivity is linked to flare-ups of the rash. And the majority of people with atopic dermatitis have a personal or family history of allergy.

Q: What allergies have been linked to atopic dermatitis?

A: Food allergies are responsible for flare-ups in about 10 percent of atopic dermatitis patients. Allergies to pollen, dust mites and dander have also been linked to atopic dermatitis.

Q: Does avoiding these allergens help?

A: If the allergens are behind the flare-ups of atopic dermatitis, yes. Avoiding substances and activities that can irritate the skin—such as soaps, detergents, cleaning solvents, chemicals, wool, nylon, plastic, animals, frequent washing with hot water and sweating—may also help. Otherwise, a person with eczema should concentrate on taking steps to prevent the areas of skin affected by the rash from becoming infected.

Q: So infection is a common problem with eczema?

A: Yes. Remember, people with atopic dermatitis may have impaired cellular immunity and may be more susceptible to infection. In addition, because atopic dermatitis is so itchy, it is hard to resist the urge to scratch it. Scratching further irritates the skin and can cause it to break open, making it more susceptible to infection. Infections require a doctor's treatment.

Q: What steps can I take to minimize the risk of infection?

A: For starters, don't scratch. You should also try to moisten your dry skin. You can do this by taking soaking baths or showers in tepid (not hot) water twice a day, patting (not rubbing) your skin dry, then applying a moisturizer—either a petroleum product such as petroleum jelly or a nonperfumed skin cream.

Q: Is there anything else I should do?

A: There are topical and oral medications, available both by prescription and over the counter, that can be used to treat some of the symptoms of atopic dermatitis. We discuss these medications in chapter 9.

ALLERGIC CONTACT DERMATITIS

Q: How does allergic contact dermatitis differ from atopic dermatitis?

A: Although both allergic contact dermatitis and atopic dermatitis involve a rash—an inflammation (*itis*) of the skin (*derm*)—there are several key differences. For one, while allergens are directly responsible for triggering atopic dermatitis only on occasion, they are always the cause of allergic contact dermatitis. For another, the allergens that trigger or worsen atopic dermatitis are generally inhaled or ingested, while the allergens that trigger allergic contact dermatitis are encountered through physical contact. And the rashes themselves may differ in appearance.

Q: **What does the allergic contact dermatitis rash look like?**

A: Generally, the rash consists of red, warm bumps or blisters, which may break and ooze. If you can picture the rash caused by poison ivy, you know what allergic contact dermatitis looks like.

Q: **So poison ivy is an allergen?**

A: No, the plant is not an allergen. But **urushiol**, the oily resin it produces, is. This resin, found in poison ivy, poison oak and poison sumac, is the most common cause of allergic contact dermatitis.

Q: **Do I have to actually come into contact with this resin in order to develop a rash?**

A: Yes. But since the resin may remain on articles of clothing that have brushed against the plant or on dogs, cats or other animals that have come into contact with the plant, it's possible to develop a rash without ever touching one of the notorious plants.

Q: **Nearly everybody I know has had poison ivy at one time or another. Yet many of them don't have any other allergies. Is it possible for people who don't have other allergies to be allergic to poison ivy?**

A: Yes. Allergic contact dermatitis can affect both allergy-prone and non-allergy-prone individuals.

Q: Why is that?

A: That's a very good question—one that brings us back to our discussion of the immune system and the mechanisms of allergy. As you'll recall, allergy occurs when the immune system mistakes a harmless substance for a harmful substance and sets out to attack it. In most instances of allergy, the body reacts by producing IgE antibodies, which bind with and neutralize allergens, triggering the immediate release of chemical mediators such as histamine from the mast cells and basophils. In the case of allergic contact dermatitis, however, the protective mechanism differs.

Allergic contact dermatitis occurs when the body's T cells, sensitized to a foreign substance, recognize it as an allergen, migrate to it and secrete mediators of their own—in this case lymphokines. These lymphokines attract phagocytes to the site. These white blood cells engulf and ingest the invading allergen, eventually resulting in the development of a rash.

Q: So the rash is a result of the body's attempt to rid itself of the allergen?

A: Yes. You'll recall from chapter 2 that the immune system's attempt to rid the body of foreign substances it sees as dangerous—whether by means of antibodies or by means of T cells—produces an inflammatory response. In the case of allergic contact dermatitis, that response takes the form of a rash.

Q: So getting back to my original question: Allergic contact dermatitis affects both allergy-prone and non-allergy-prone individuals because . . . ?

A: It occurs by a mechanism that does not involve an inherited tendency to produce IgE antibodies. It simply involves sensitization to a substance.

Q: So there's no way to tell who will get poison ivy?

A: Not really. As we just said, the only mechanism involved is sensitization. No matter what your sensitivity, if you've never come into contact with poison ivy, you won't develop a rash on your first exposure. But after that, there's no way of predicting. Some people may become sensitized after a few encounters with the plant; others may become sensitized only after years of exposure; and still others may never become sensitized, no matter how many times they encounter the "leaves of three."

Q: I heard somewhere that poison ivy can also cause problems if it's inhaled. Is that true?

A: It's true, although it's uncommon. Most reactions to poison ivy are the result of skin contact with the resin. But some people try to get rid of the plants by burning them. While this does destroy the plants, it sends their resin into the air. From there, it can either come into contact with large areas of skin, causing a widespread rash, or be inhaled, causing an internal reaction. Needless to say, this is not the optimum way to get rid of poison ivy plants. A standard herbicide is much safer.

Q: Is it true that the poison ivy rash can be spread by scratching?

A: No. The blisters do not contain any resin, and it is the resin that causes the rash. It is true, however, that if you touch another part of your body while the resin is still on your hands, you can develop the rash on the area you touch. This makes it important to wash your hands thoroughly as soon as possible after you come in contact with poison ivy.

Q: How long after touching the resin does the rash appear?

A: Generally, one to two days. Poison ivy and other forms of allergic contact dermatitis are examples of delayed hypersensitivity. This means the allergic reaction does not occur immediately on contact with the allergen, as it does when IgE antibodies are involved (as in cases of allergic rhinitis). In the case of allergic contact dermatitis, contact occurs on one day, and the rash breaks out one to two days later.

Q: How long does the allergic contact dermatitis rash last?

A: Allergic contact dermatitis can be acute or chronic. Acute reactions, such as those to poison ivy, generally last for several weeks. Chronic reactions can occur when there is repeated or continuous exposure to the allergen and, thus, can last until the exposure comes to an end.

Q: What allergens other than poison ivy cause allergic contact dermatitis?

A: Common causes of allergic contact dermatitis include nail polish, hair dyes and permanent solutions, shampoos, cosmetics, perfumes, underarm deodorants, formaldehyde (which is common in fabric and wood products), clothing dyes, leather, glue, plastic, cement, preservatives such as ethylenediamine (used in topical creams and lotions), metals such as nickel (used in jewelry) and latex.

Q: I thought you said in the last chapter that latex causes respiratory allergies?

A: Latex, a natural, milky sap from the tropical rubber tree, can cause respiratory allergies when it is airborne. (You'll recall that the latex allergen attaches itself to the cornstarch powder inside latex gloves and becomes airborne.) But latex can also cause allergic contact dermatitis, hives or even anaphylactic shock.

Q: Which reaction is the most common?

A: The most common reaction to latex is allergic contact dermatitis.

Q: Where does a person come into contact with latex?

A: We already discussed the fact that latex is used in surgical gloves. It is also used in catheters (hollow, flexible tubes that allow fluids to pass in and out of the body during treatments and tests), dishwashing gloves, rubber bands, balloons and condoms.

Q: You said earlier that the incidence of latex allergy is highest among health-care workers. Is allergic contact dermatitis a problem in other professions as well?

A: Yes. It's a fairly common complaint in many industries; in some factories, the incidence among workers is estimated at between 8 and 12 percent. Chromium salt often causes allergic contact dermatitis in people who work with cement or in the tanning, dyeing or printing industries, for example, while construction workers who handle wallboard are occasionally exposed to formaldehyde.

Q: How do doctors determine what is causing a rash?

A: A person's history—particularly information about her occupation, hobbies, clothing, cosmetics, jewelry and outdoor exposure—is extremely important in diagnosing allergic contact dermatitis. A physical exam can also yield important information. If the rash appears on the edges of the scalp and forehead, for example, it might mean the person is allergic to hair dye or hair lotion or even to something in her hatband. If it appears on the earlobes, it might mean she is allergic to nickel or some other metal in her earrings. Doctors also use the patch test, which we described in chapter 3, to determine which allergen is causing allergic contact dermatitis.

Q: Does avoiding the allergen end the problem?

A: Yes and no. Avoiding the allergen will prevent future eruptions of the rash, but any existing rash must run its course.

Q: What is that course?

A: The rash begins with the reddening and swelling of the affected area, followed by the development of small, itchy blisters and bumps. The blisters fill with clear fluid, then burst, revealing raw skin susceptible to bacteria and infection. The skin then gradually becomes less inflamed as it heals.

Q: Is there any treatment?

A: Yes, there are medications available to relieve the itching and help speed the healing process. We discuss these treatments in chapter 9.

6 FOOD, DRUG AND INSECT ALLERGIES

Q: I thought we covered food, drug and insect allergies earlier. What more is there to know about them?

A: Plenty. While it's true that allergies to foods, drugs and insects can trigger the respiratory and skin reactions we discussed in chapters 4 and 5, they can also provoke other reactions, including anaphylaxis. In fact, because these allergens are consumed or are introduced directly into the body by means of injection, sting or bite, they can travel throughout the body with ease, making body-wide, or systemic, reactions more common with them than with other allergens.

Q: Refresh my memory. What is anaphylaxis?

A: Anaphylaxis is the most severe type of allergic reaction: It can affect a person's entire body. Symptoms range from a mild case of systemic hives, accompanied by itching, flushing and angioedema, to cramping and diarrhea, swelling of the larynx (voice box), difficulty breathing, a reduction in blood pressure and, occasionally, shock, circulatory collapse and death.

FOOD ALLERGY

Q: Now that I think of it, I hear a lot of people say that they're allergic to this food or that food. Is food allergy common?

A: Although many people believe that they are allergic to foods, the actual number of people with food allergies is relatively low. Experts estimate that only 2 percent of adults and from 2 to 8 percent of children are truly allergic to foods.

Q: Then why do so many people say they are allergic to foods?

A: Many people are not actually allergic to foods but instead are intolerant of them. And food intolerance can cause symptoms similar to those of food allergy.

Q: What are the symptoms of food allergy?

A: As we've said, food allergy can provoke hives, trigger asthma, cause allergic rhinitis and allergic conjunctivitis, exacerbate eczema and lead to anaphylaxis. When food allergy affects the mouth, it can provoke what is known as **oral allergy syndrome**: It can make the lips tingle, itch and swell and, occasionally, make the throat tighten. And when food allergy affects the gastrointestinal tract, it can cause cramping, bloating, nausea, vomiting and diarrhea.

Intolerance

Q: Now can you tell me more about food intolerance? What is it, and what are its symptoms?

A: Food intolerance is an abnormal reaction to a food or food additive (such as a preservative or dye) that is not caused by the immune system. In other words, it is not caused by the joining of an allergen and an immunoglobulin E antibody. Food intolerance is often caused by an inability to metabolize, or break down, certain foods or by a sensitivity to druglike chemicals naturally contained in foods.

Q: Could you give me some examples?

A: Certainly. Many people are intolerant of **lactose**, the sugar in milk. This is because their bodies lack lactase, the enzyme needed to break down and digest lactose. As a result, these people experience stomach cramps and diarrhea when they drink milk. They are not allergic to milk, but they experience symptoms typical of food allergy.

Likewise, some people get headaches when they eat cheese or chocolate. This is a reaction to druglike chemicals in the foods—tyramine in the case of cheese and phenylethylamine in the case of chocolate. (Even though headache is not a typical allergy symptom, some people recognize a link between foods they eat and headaches that follow and assign the blame to allergy.)

Q: What other symptoms can be caused by food intolerance?

A: Food intolerance can provoke nausea, vomiting and other gastrointestinal symptoms common to allergy; nasal symptoms reminiscent of allergic rhinitis; and a rash around the mouth. In some people, food intolerance manifests itself with an **anaphylactoid reaction**, which is similar to an anaphylactic reaction but is not triggered by IgE antibodies. In an anaphylactoid reaction, mast cells release histamine and other mediators, as they do in a true anaphylactic reaction, but it is not known what triggers this release. Regardless of the trigger, however, anaphylactoid reactions can be serious, even life-threatening. They require the same emergency treatment as anaphylactic reactions.

Q: What type of treatment is that?

A: Anaphylactic and anaphylactoid reactions are treated with **epinephrine**, a hormonelike drug that counteracts anaphylaxis by opening airways and increasing blood pressure and blood flow to the heart. This potent drug, which we discuss in more detail in chapter 9, is given by injection as soon as possible after the reaction has started. Doctors often prescribe user-friendly premeasured syringes of epinephrine to people at risk for anaphylaxis and advise them to carry the syringes with them when they are in situations that place them at risk.

Q: Getting back to food intolerance, are any other symptoms possible?

A: Yes. Migraines and an exacerbation of arthritis have also been attributed to food intolerance.

Q: Is food intolerance common?

A: It is far more common than food allergy. Approximately 20 percent of people surveyed in a 1994 British study said they have experienced some type of adverse reaction to food. Other surveys have placed the figure at 25 percent. Bear in mind, however, that these surveys are subjective: They indicate only the number of people who think they have a problem with food, be it allergy or intolerance. Still, it is estimated that about 80 percent of African-Americans are lactose-intolerant, as are many people of Mediterranean or Hispanic origin. And other problems are also relatively common.

Common Food Allergens

Q: Speaking of common problems, which foods are the most common causes of food allergy?

A: The most common causes of food allergy in children are milk, eggs, wheat, peanuts, nuts, soy, fish and shellfish. In adults, peanuts, nuts, fish and shellfish are the prime culprits.

Q: The children's list is longer than the adults' list. Why is that?

A: Generally, food allergies first become apparent in childhood. Many such reactions are outgrown, often within a child's first three years. But allergies to peanuts, nuts, fish and shellfish tend to persist throughout life.

Q: I've heard that people have died after eating peanuts. Are peanuts particularly dangerous?

A: Peanut allergy can be serious. In fact, the protein in this legume has been responsible for more food allergy deaths than any other allergen, in part because peanuts are often hidden as ingredients in other foods. Peanuts are often used in baked goods, candy and Chinese and Thai foods, but their use is not always obvious. Some Chinese restaurants have been known to use peanut butter to seal their egg rolls, for example. So as you can imagine, it's very important for people with peanut allergy to read food labels and to ask questions of food preparers. And since peanut allergy often manifests itself as anaphylaxis, peanut-allergic people should carry epinephrine.

One final word on peanuts: People who are allergic to them may also be allergic to other legumes, such as peas, beans, soybeans, chickpeas and lentils.

Q: Why is that?

A: It's because of a phenomenon known as **cross-reactivity**. Cross-reactivity occurs when IgE antibodies react to a substance that is similar to the allergen that caused their creation. This reaction can occur whether or not a person has had prior exposure to the similar substance.

Q: Wait a minute. I thought prior exposure was a necessary ingredient for an allergic reaction. Are you saying it isn't?

A: No. We're saying that in some instances, a person can experience an allergic reaction to a substance to which he has not been exposed if he *has* been exposed to a similar substance. The exposure element is still there; it simply refers to the original allergen.

Q: How similar do substances have to be to cause cross-reactivity? If I'm allergic to corn, do I run the risk of being allergic to all vegetables?

A: No. The similarities run deeper than that. People do not develop allergies to all vegetables, all fruits, all nuts or all meats. They generally develop allergies to vegetables, fruits or nuts that are in the same plant family or fish, shellfish or meats that are in the same animal family.

Peanuts, for example, are in the legume family. As we said, people who are allergic to peanuts may also be allergic to other legumes. Likewise, people allergic to other legumes may be also be allergic to peanuts. This does not mean, however, that a peanut-allergic person will automatically be allergic to all—or even any— other legumes. It simply means that he is more likely to be allergic to other legumes than someone without peanut allergy.

Q: Could you give me some other examples?

A: Certainly. Let's start with shellfish, fish and nuts, which, along with legumes, are the most common causes of food allergy.

If you're allergic to one food in any of the following categories (marked with bullets), there's a good chance that you might be allergic to other foods in that category:

Shellfish

- Crustaceans: crab, crayfish, lobster, shrimp
- Mollusks: abalones, clams, escargots, mussels, octopus, oysters, scallops, squid

Fish

- Centrarchidae: black bass, crappie, sunfish
- Clupeidae: herring, sardines, shad
- Esocidae: muskellunge, pickerel, pike
- Gadidae: cod, haddock, pollack, scrod
- Pleuronectidae: flounder, halibut
- Salmonidae: grayling, salmon, trout, whitefish

- Scombridae: mackerel, tuna
- Serranidae: grouper, rockfish, white bass

Nuts

- Beeches: beechnuts, chestnuts
- Cashews: cashews, mangoes, pistachios (mangoes are not nuts but are in the same plant family as cashews and pistachios)
- Walnuts: black walnuts, butternuts, English walnuts, hickory nuts, pecans

Because almonds are in the plum family, people who are allergic to almonds may also be allergic to plums, prunes, peaches, nectarines, apricots and cherries. Likewise, people allergic to one or more of these fruits may also be allergic to almonds.

 Are there any other allergenic food families I should know about?

There certainly are. Here are some common ones:

- Cereals: barley, corn, hominy, malt, oats, rice, rye, sorghum, sugarcane, wheat
- Citrus: grapefruit, kumquats, lemons, limes, oranges, tangelos, tangerines
- Gourds: cantaloupe, casaba, cucumbers, honeydew, pumpkin, summer squash, watermelon, winter squash
- Lilies: asparagus, chives, garlic, leeks, onions, shallots
- Mustards: broccoli, brussels sprouts, cabbage, cauliflower, collards, horseradish, kale, kohlrabi, mustard, radishes, rutabagas, turnips, watercress
- Nightshades: bell peppers, chili peppers, eggplant, potatoes, tobacco, tomatoes
- Parsley: anise, caraway, carrots, celeriac, celery, coriander, dill, fennel, parsley, parsnips

Cross-reactions can also occur between plant families. For example, researchers have found that people who are allergic to avocados, bananas, water chestnuts or kiwifruit are more likely to be allergic to latex than other people. Likewise, people who are allergic to latex are more likely to be allergic to one of these foods. And eating cantaloupe, bananas, watermelon or honeydew or drinking chamomile tea has been found to intensify the allergic reaction to ragweed pollen in some people.

Q: **Wait a minute! I thought plants had to be from the same plant family to cross-react. How can plants from different families cross-react?**

A: Most cross-reactivity does occur within the same plant family, but some plants from different families contain identical proteins. And generally, a person develops allergies to proteins contained in foods—not to foods in general.

Q: **So if I react to milk, I'm really reacting not to the milk itself but to a protein in the milk?**

A: Yes. In fact, milk contains several allergenic proteins, the primary ones being **casein** and the **whey** proteins beta-lactoglobulin and alpha-lactalbumin. Likewise, if you're allergic to eggs, you're probably allergic to the allergenic protein **albumin**, or **ovalbumin**, which is found in egg whites. It's important to know the names of these proteins, since they are often used in processed foods.

Q: **Do the labels of processed foods identify these proteins as milk or egg products?**

A: That depends on the food in question. The Nutrition Labeling and Education Act, which went into effect in 1994, requires manufacturers to refer to casein as a milk derivative in the ingredient lists of foods that claim to be nondairy, such as coffee creamers. But while the act also requires manufacturers to list the sources of proteins used as flavors and flavor enhancers in foods, it's up to the consumer to know if those proteins come from milk, eggs or some other food to which he is allergic. So it helps to know the names of the proteins.

Q: It probably helps to read food labels, too. Right?

A: Absolutely. Food labels should be required reading for anyone with an allergy or intolerance to a food or food additive. The new labeling law requires manufacturers to list Food and Drug Administration–certified color additives by name on ingredient lists and to include ingredient lists for all foods that have more than one ingredient. (In the past, so-called standardized foods were not required to include lists of ingredients.)

Common Food Additive Allergens

Q: You said the law now requires food labels to list food colorings by name. Do colorings present a problem?

A: For some people, yes. Food dyes, along with other food additives such as preservatives and flavor enhancers, can cause allergic reactions, exacerbate allergic conditions or prompt intolerance reactions.

Q: Could you list some common problem additives and tell me what they do?

A: Certainly. The dye **tartrazine** (FD&C Yellow No. 5), which is used to color foods and medicines, has been shown to cause asthma flare-ups in some people and has also been linked to hives. Benzoates, butylated hydroxytoluene (BHT) and hydroxyanisole—which are used as preservatives in ready-made foods, breads, milk, fats, oils, margarine, mayonnaise and soft drinks—have been linked to hives. And **sulfites**, preservatives used in processed foods and beverages such as processed shellfish and mushrooms, potato chips, dried fruits and wine, have been linked to a host of allergy-like reactions, including rhinitis, hives, asthma flare-ups and anaphylaxis.

Q: You know, I never really thought of all of the different items we ingest and the various problems they can open us up to. Wouldn't we head off a lot of trouble if we limited what we eat to a few safe things?

A: No, we wouldn't. The more we eat of a specific food, the more we are exposed to that food. And exposure, as you know, is one of the key factors in developing allergy. After all, young children, who are continuously exposed to cow's milk, have a higher prevalence of milk allergy than do adults. And in Japan, where soy is commonly eaten, there is a higher prevalence of soy allergy. Allergy-prone people who restrict their diets to a few foods may ultimately sensitize themselves to those foods by repeated exposure.

But the main reason we should not severely limit our diets to prevent food allergy is that it's unhealthy: We need to eat well-balanced diets. We may need to eliminate certain foods from our diets if we suffer from food allergy or intolerance, but widespread deprivation is rarely necessary and often harmful.

Q: Harmful?

A: Yes—particularly for children. In a 1994 study, published in the *Archives of Pediatrics & Adolescent Medicine*, 11 children under three years old, whose parents removed an average of eight foods from their diets "to take care of" allergies, experienced low rates of growth and weight gain that put them at risk for brain damage and other developmental problems. And in Britain, a nationwide survey of children ages 5 to 11 found that children perceived by their parents as food-intolerant were more than one-half inch shorter than other children their age.

Even adults may suffer from strict elimination diets, according to a review in the November 25, 1992, *Journal of the American Medical Association.* The review warned that elimination diets may lead to malnutrition and/or eating disorders, especially if they include a large number of foods or are used for extended periods of time.

Q: OK, I take back my suggestion. But am I right to assume that we should at least stop eating foods that we know cause problems?

A: Yes. In fact, avoidance is the only way to prevent food-triggered allergic reactions. Desensitization, also known as **immunotherapy** or allergy shots, has not yet been proven effective against food allergens. Thus, it's important to be aware of food allergies and to avoid eating foods or food additives to which you are allergic or for which you have an intolerance. This means you need to read food labels and ask questions, so you'll be able to recognize potential sources of hidden food allergens. Be particularly cautious when in restaurants, where foods may contain multiple ingredients but the ingredients are not generally listed.

But since even the most careful person may inadvertently eat a food to which he is allergic, food-allergic people—particularly those who have experienced anaphylactic reactions to foods in the past—should carry a kit containing epinephrine and learn how to inject themselves in case of emergency.

The importance of this emergency measure was brought home in a 1992 Johns Hopkins University School of Medicine study, which found that 13 children suffered fatal or near-fatal allergic reactions to foods they had consumed unwittingly. The children and their parents were all aware of the allergies, but not of their potential seriousness. As a result, they were unprepared to take emergency action when the children accidentally ate foods containing ingredients to which they were allergic. The study authors warned that hidden allergens may become even more of a problem in the future, as more and more people turn to processed foods. And it appears that genetically engineered foods may pose problems as well.

Q: What are genetically engineered foods?

A: Genetically engineered foods are foods whose genes have been altered to include or exclude certain proteins, enzymes or other building blocks in order to change a trait, or traits, of the original foods.

Q: How do these foods pose problems for food-allergic people?

A: By transferring allergenic proteins from one food to another. A study published in the March 14, 1996, *New England Journal of Medicine* found that eight of nine people allergic to Brazil nuts showed signs of allergic reaction when they were exposed to extracts of soybeans genetically engineered to contain a protein found in Brazil nuts.

Q: Is this a common problem?

A: Not yet. Most genetically engineered food products are created by adding genes from nonfoods—substances that are not allergenic—to foods. Only a small percentage of these foods use proteins known to cause allergic reactions. But according to an editorial that accompanied the Brazil nut study, there is still a "big unknown" when companies experiment with such technology, and "unexpected, unpleasant consequences can result."

DRUG ALLERGY

Q: That's progress for you! Speaking of progress, what about drugs? What kinds of allergies can they cause?

A: Like foods, drugs can cause a variety of adverse effects, including allergies, intolerance, side effects, overdoses and drug interactions. The majority of these adverse reactions—more than 90 percent by most estimates—are not caused by allergy. But as with foods, many people attribute the adverse reactions they experience after taking drugs to allergy, whether or not allergy is the actual cause. This is because the symptoms can be similar: Drug allergy can cause anaphylaxis, while other types of adverse drug reactions can cause anaphylactoid reactions. Similarly, both drug allergy and other types of drug reactions commonly cause hives and rashes.

Q: I know you said adverse reactions to drugs are more common than allergies to drugs, but how common is drug allergy?

A: Experts estimate that about 5 percent of the population is allergic to a drug.

Q: Which drugs cause the most problems?

A: The biggest villain, ironically, is penicillin, an antibiotic that has saved countless lives. Anaphylactic reactions reportedly occur in from 1 to 5 of every 10,000 doses of penicillin given. And 75 percent of deaths from anaphylaxis in the United States are attributed to penicillin. But hives and angioedema are more common reactions. Fever can also occur as an allergic reaction to penicillin.

Hives, angioedema, fever and anaphylaxis may also result from penicillin-related antibiotics such as ampicillin and amoxicillin and, occasionally, from cephalosporins, which are chemically related to penicillin. People who are allergic to penicillin are almost always allergic to amoxicillin and ampicillin and are occasionally allergic to cephalosporins, including cephalexin (Keflex), cefaclor (Ceclor), cefuroxime (Ceftin) and cefixime (Suprax).

Another class of drugs that commonly cause allergic reactions is the **sulfonamides**, or sulfa drugs. These drugs are used to fight bacterial infection. They include sulfamethoxazole (Bactrim, Gantanol, Septra), sulfisoxazole (Gantrisin) and diuretics that contain sulfonamides—chlorothiazide (Diuril), chlorthalidone (Thalitone), hydroflumethiazide (Diucardin), methyclothiazide (Enduron), hydrochlorothiazide (Esidrix, HydroDIURIL, Oretic) and indapamide (Lozol).

Q: Do any other drugs commonly cause allergic reactions?

A: Many drugs can cause allergic reactions. Penicillin, penicillin-related drugs and sulfa drugs are the most common culprits, but other drugs have been known to cause allergic reactions with some regularity.

Other drugs known to cause *anaphylaxis* include:

- hormones such as insulin
- chymopapain, an enzyme used to treat ruptured or herniated disks in the vertebrae
- muscle relaxants used during the early stages of general anesthesia
- streptokinase, an enzyme used to dissolve blood clots and treat circulatory system disorders
- vaccines such as the measles-mumps-rubella vaccine

Other drugs known to cause *hives* or *rashes* include:

- barbiturates, a class of drugs used as sedatives
- iodides, compounds that include iodine
- phenolphthalein, found in some laxative preparations

Drugs, other than sulfa drugs, known to cause *skin reactions after sun exposure* (**photoallergic reactions**) include:

- griseofulvin (Fulvicin, Grifulvin, Grisactin), an antibiotic
- psoralens, chemical compounds used in skin tanning products, perfumes, colognes and hair creams as well as in drugs used to treat skin diseases such as psoriasis and vitiligo

Drugs that exacerbate *eczema* include:

- neomycin sulfate, an antibiotic found in Cortisporin, NeoDecadron and Neosporin
- benzocaine, a topical anesthetic
- bacitracin, an antibiotic found in Cortisporin, Neosporin and Polysporin

Q: **What about aspirin? I thought a lot of people were allergic to aspirin.**

A: Aspirin and other nonsteroidal anti-inflammatory drugs (NSAIDs), including ibuprofen (Motrin, Advil, Nuprin) and indomethacin, do indeed cause problems for a number of people. But the reactions these medications cause are known as **pseudoallergic reactions**: They resemble allergic reactions but are not actually caused by allergy.

Aspirin and NSAIDs can severely exacerbate asthma, especially in people with nasal polyps or chronic sinusitis. In fact, it is estimated that 1 in 10 asthma patients is sensitive to aspirin and NSAIDs. These drugs can also cause hives and provoke attacks of rhinitis. Experts are not yet sure what mechanism is involved in these reactions. They simply know that the mechanism is not allergic in nature. It's a problem of drug intolerance.

Q: Do any other drugs widely cause intolerance problems?

A: Yes. Drugs that directly stimulate mast cells or basophils to release histamine or other mediators can cause anaphylactoid reactions and other problems. These include drugs containing opium and x-ray dyes, or **radiocontrast media**. (These dyes are used to help radiologists see organs being studied in x-rays, computed axial tomography or CAT scans, myelograms and angiography.) These drugs are known to trigger anaphylactoid reactions.

Drugs that directly stimulate the mast cells cause other problems. The antibiotic vancomycin has been associated with itching, swelling and angioedema over the upper body. And angiotensin-converting enzyme (ACE) inhibitors, drugs used to control high blood pressure, are known to generate a nonallergic rash, a dry cough and, occasionally, angioedema.

Q: Should people who are intolerant of these drugs avoid them?

A: Of course. Drug intolerance, like drug allergy, can provoke severe reactions. Anaphylactoid reactions can be just as serious as anaphylactic reactions; they are simply triggered by different mechanisms. Whenever possible, people who are drug-allergic or drug-intolerant should avoid the drugs to which they react. And as with food allergy or intolerance, avoidance means reading labels and asking questions.

Q: Why is that?

A: For two reasons: (1) Some medications contain more than one ingredient; and (2) some medications are chemically similar to other medications to which a person may be allergic.

Q: Could you give me some examples of medications that contain more than one ingredient?

A: We've already seen several. We noted, for instance, that diuretics containing sulfonamides can be allergenic, even though diuretics themselves generally don't provoke reactions. Likewise, we saw that certain drug combinations that contain neomycin sulfite and bacitracin can provoke allergy even though other ingredients in the preparations are not generally allergenic.

Even over-the-counter drugs are not immune to this phenomenon. If you're aspirin-intolerant, chances are you'll reach for acetaminophen (Tylenol) rather than aspirin when you have a headache. But you might inadvertently ingest aspirin when you attempt to relieve cold symptoms with an over-the-counter cold remedy: Many of them contain aspirin.

Q: I hadn't thought of that. What about medications that are chemically similar to other medications?

A: Penicillin is the best example. As we've seen, people who are allergic to penicillin are often also allergic to related drugs such as ampicillin and amoxicillin. And because there is a chemical similarity between penicillin and cephalosporins, penicillin-allergic people often react to cephalosporins as well.

Q: But what happens if a penicillin-allergic person needs an antibiotic?

A: In most cases, the doctor will substitute an antibiotic that is not chemically similar to penicillin. The same holds true for other drug allergies. In some instances, however, substitution may not be possible. The problem drug may be the best—

or even the only—product available to treat a condition. In these cases, the doctor may put the allergic person through a rapid desensitization program designed to make treatment with the drug feasible. Bear in mind, however, that this is done only in extreme cases. The standard method for dealing with allergies to drugs, as for allergies to foods and other allergens, is avoidance.

INSECT ALLERGY

Q: **I hate insects, so I really wouldn't mind avoiding them. Which ones cause allergies?**

A: As we mentioned in chapter 5, although biting insects such as the mosquito can cause allergic reactions, stinging insects from the Hymenoptera class are the prime culprits. This class includes **vespids** such as the yellow jacket, hornet and wasp and **apids** such as the honeybee and bumblebee. It also includes the fire ant, which lives in the southeastern and south-central United States—especially along the Gulf coast.

Q: **Does any one of these insects cause more problems than the others?**

A: Yes. In most parts of the United States, yellow jackets are the principal cause of allergic reactions to insect stings.

Q: **Why is that?**

A: It's the nature of the beast—or should we say the nature of the bee. Yellow jackets nest in the ground or in walls and are easily disturbed by lawn mowing, gardening and other outdoor activities. And because they feed on sugar, they are attracted to food and garbage. In addition, these insects are capable of inflicting multiple stings, unlike honeybees, which sting only once and are not very aggressive.

Q: Speaking of aggressive, do killer bees pose any special problems?

A: Africanized honeybees—the so-called killer bees— entered the Southwest several years ago and have slowly been traveling northward. Their venom is no more allergenic or toxic (poisonous) than the venom of the standard honeybee, but they are much more aggressive and may sting en masse.

Q: How many people are allergic to stinging insects?

A: It is estimated that more than 2 million Americans are allergic to stinging insects. More than 500,000 people enter hospital emergency rooms each year for treatment of stings, and 40 to 150 people die as the result of allergic reactions to insect stings.

Q: But that's the extreme. What are the most common symptoms of insect allergy, and how do they differ from the typical sting reaction?

A: Most people experience localized pain, swelling and redness at the site of a sting—a reaction that lasts for several hours. This is not an allergic reaction; it is simply the body's way of responding to the toxins in the insect venom. In some allergic people, however, this reaction is more extensive. The swelling may extend over a large area, can last for several days and may be accompanied by fatigue and nausea.

In other people, the allergy manifests itself as anaphylaxis. The most common symptoms are generalized hives, angioedema and flushing. Less common but more serious symptoms include breathing difficulties, dizziness, a drop in blood pressure, nausea, cramps or diarrhea and, in extreme cases, shock and cardiac arrest.

Q: Is there any way to know if I'll experience an allergic reaction to a sting?

A: The most important tool in diagnosing insect allergy is medical history. If you've experienced a large local reaction, developed hives on various parts of your body or experienced other symptoms of anaphylaxis after being stung, it is likely that you are allergic to the insect that stung you. Skin tests and blood tests are available to confirm your allergy and identify the insect that causes the reaction. But these tests are generally not performed unless a person has a history of reacting to stings.

Q: Why is that?

A: For one thing, the skin tests—which are the most sensitive of the two types of tests—can provoke allergic reactions. For another, most people try to avoid stinging insects whether they are allergic or not. They don't need the allergy diagnosis to begin first-line treatment: avoidance.

Q: Point made. We'll stick with the history. Let's say I've had a large local reaction to a bee sting. Will I react the same way the next time I'm stung?

A: It's quite possible. People who have had large local reactions to stings—and nothing more—generally have similar reactions after subsequent stings. Their risk of anaphylaxis, however, is relatively low; studies place it at less than 5 percent.

Q: What about people who have experienced anaphylactic reactions to stings?

A: These people are at risk for experiencing anaphylactic reactions to subsequent stings.

Q: Is there anything these people can do to prevent this from happening?

A: There is. They can minimize their exposure to stinging insects and keep epinephrine on hand for emergency use. They can also consider desensitization. Venom immunotherapy is very effective in preventing future episodes of anaphylaxis. It reduces the risk of recurrent anaphylaxis from between 50 and 60 percent to about 10 percent after two years and to 2 percent after three to five years, according to a review in the August 25, 1994, *New England Journal of Medicine*. We have more to say about immunotherapy in chapter 10.

Q: Good. In the meantime, how can I minimize my exposure to stinging insects?

A: Here are some tips:

- Wear shoes, slacks and long sleeves in grassy areas and fields.
- Wear gloves when gardening.
- Avoid wearing scented cosmetics, perfumes and hair sprays. (Bees are attracted to the scents.)
- Wear dark-, drab- or neutral-colored clothing. (Bees are attracted to bright colors.)
- Take care when cooking and eating outdoors.
- Do not swat at bees.

Q: Didn't you say that bites from insects can also cause allergic reactions?

A: Yes. Biting insects such as mosquitoes and fleas deposit salivary gland secretions in the body when they bite. And people can develop allergies to these secretions.

Q: How serious are allergic reactions to these secretions?

A: Although there have been incidents when anaphylaxis occurred as the result of a deerfly, kissing bug or bedbug bite, insect bites rarely cause anaphylaxis. The most common reaction to these bites is a large local reaction.

7 IRRITANTS, SICK BUILDINGS AND CLINICAL ECOLOGY

Q: We seem to have addressed the major allergens, but I still have some questions. I hear a lot of people attribute a lot of different symptoms to what they call environmental allergies—allergies to things in the environment such as air pollution, chemicals and even the buildings they work in. Are such allergies possible?

A: There is no question that many things in our environment can make us sick. Tobacco smoke can cause lung cancer; industrial chemicals can burn our skin or, when released into the air, cause breathing difficulties; gasoline and similar products can give us headaches when inhaled; and household chemicals can make us nauseated. These symptoms are real, and they are indeed caused by exposure to things in the environment. But they are not caused by the binding of an allergen to an immunoglobulin E antibody, which is, you'll remember, the classic definition of allergy. Consequently, these problems are not allergies, according to the conventional definition.

Q: Then why do people call them allergies?

A: For several reasons. For one thing, the symptoms may be similar to those of allergies. For another, the link between the environmental substance and the symptoms may be obvious. As you may recall from our discussion of food and drug intolerances, many people notice a link between eating a food or taking a drug and experiencing symptoms. They automatically assume that they are allergic to the food or drug in question when they are actually intolerant of it or sensitive to it. Likewise, people can be intolerant of or sensitive to (or allergic to) things in the air.

These intolerances or sensitivities can provoke some type of physiological symptom or symptoms, and people may simply assume these symptoms are the result of allergy.

Finally, there is a group of doctors who practice what is known as **clinical ecology**, or **environmental medicine**. These doctors entertain a much wider definition of allergy—one that ascribes a wide range of symptoms to exposure to numerous common substances in the environment. Under their definition, these reactions can indeed be called allergies.

Q: **I want to know a little bit more about clinical ecology, but first I'd like to know more about substances in the environment that can cause problems. Could you list a few?**

A: A large number of common substances act as irritants. They include tobacco smoke; household chemicals such as disinfectants, ammonia, chlorine, floor wax and paint; personal care products such as perfumes, powders, shampoos and hair sprays; the smell of heating or cooking gas; fumes from the chemicals in building materials, carpeting and dry-cleaned clothing; pesticides and insecticides; components of air pollution, including sulfur dioxide, diesel fuel exhaust, automobile exhaust and emissions from factories; and fumes from brushfires, burning leaves and garbage.

These irritants can trigger asthma attacks, cause flare-ups of allergic nasal congestion and increase the severity of allergy attacks. They can also cause problems of their own, including headaches, fatigue and nausea.

Q: **How can these irritants trigger asthma attacks or make allergy symptoms worse?**

A: Irritants are just that—irritants. They can irritate the lungs, which starts the asthma cycle of bronchospasms, mucus production and airway inflammation, or they can irritate the nose, which prompts inflammation. In fact, people with allergies are often affected by small amounts of irritants that others notice only in high doses. They may become quite sick upon inhaling tobacco smoke, for example, even though the smoke itself is nonallergenic (the leaf, however, is not).

Q: Backing up to the list of irritants, you mentioned chemical fumes from building materials. Can buildings themselves make people sick?

A: No—but the irritants, pollutants and allergens in them can. No doubt you've heard the term **sick building syndrome**, which refers to a situation in which a number of people in a building experience a variety of symptoms when they're in the building. These symptoms can include irritation or dryness of the eyes, throat and skin, headaches, a burning nose, nausea, dizziness, respiratory infections, mental fatigue and confusion. The syndrome commonly occurs in new, energy-efficient office buildings—buildings that are sealed and use recirculated air. Because these buildings are sealed, fumes from carpeting, furniture, building materials, paint, paper office supplies, copy machines, hair sprays and cleaning products, as well as bacteria, germs and allergens, continue to circulate through the air, triggering a variety of symptoms.

Q: I was aware of the problems caused by air pollution, but I didn't realize there are so many potential problems with indoor air. Is this why some people say they're allergic to the 20th century?

A: It's one of them, yes. A growing number of people believe they suffer from a condition they call **multiple chemical sensitivity**, or 20th-century disease. These people experience various reactions to a wide range of environmental chemicals— chemicals they are exposed to in both indoor and outdoor air.

Q: What types of symptoms do they experience?

A: Symptoms ascribed to multiple chemical sensitivity include confusion, memory loss, moodiness, depression, breathing difficulties, irritation, fatigue, anxiety, headaches and muscle pain. These symptoms may vary from person to person.

Q: Are these symptoms the result of allergy?

A: No. There are several theories about the cause of this controversial condition, but allergy is not among them—at least not allergy as it's traditionally defined. Some clinical ecologists do, however, attribute chemical sensitivity to a malfunction of the immune system. They believe that either the number of T cells is reduced or that their ability to function is impaired, so they can no longer control B cell production of antibodies. Without this control, the theory goes, the B cells cannot distinguish harmless allergens or even foods from toxic chemicals or bacteria and viruses.

Q: Is this theory widely accepted?

A: Not by mainstream medicine. In fact, mainstream medicine is not very accepting of clinical ecology in general because many of the theories, tests and treatments are not scientifically proven.

Q: Before we go into more detail, what exactly are the theories behind clinical ecology?

A: Clinical ecology holds that prolonged overexposure to one or more substances in the environment leads to a sensitivity, or allergy. This sensitivity, in turn, can make a person sensitive to a number of other environmental factors.

Q: What types of environmental factors trigger this sensitivity, and what symptoms do they trigger?

A: According to clinical ecologists, the triggers include the substances that cause sick building syndrome as well as substances such as air pollutants, food additives, numerous foods, viral infections, fungal infections and even water.

Symptoms can include acne, arthritis, behavior disorders, chronic fatigue, gastrointestinal problems, hypertension, hyperactivity, learning disabilities, schizophrenia, the symptoms ascribed to multiple chemical sensitivity and a host of other problems.

Q: **How do traditional doctors explain these symptoms?**

A: That depends on the symptom. Some of them are attributed to known diseases; some are the result of true allergic conditions; and still others are conditions in their own right. According to a position paper issued by the American Academy of Allergy, Asthma and Immunology, "There is no clear evidence that many of the symptoms noted . . . are related to allergy, sensitivity, toxicity or any other type of reaction from foods, water, chemicals, pollutants, viruses and bacteria in the context presented."

Q: **But clinical ecologists must have some reason for linking the symptoms to sensitivity. Do they do any type of testing?**

A: Yes, they do. But some of the tests they use to diagnose sensitivity are controversial. These include cytotoxic tests, provocation-neutralization and multiple blood tests on assorted aspects of the immune system. (You'll recall we discussed these tests back in chapter 3.) Traditional allergy tests, such as prick tests, intradermal tests and radioallergosorbent tests, may also be used.

Q: **If clinical ecologists uncover a sensitivity, how do they treat it?**

A: The hallmark of treatment is avoidance of the substance that causes the sensitivity. But since the theory holds that people often have many such sensitivities, treatment can require major changes in the environment and lifestyle, including a highly restricted diet and alterations to homes and working environments. Treatment may also include low-dose injections or under-the-tongue administration of allergen solutions—solutions that may include chemicals as well as conventional allergens. Clinical studies have not found this type of treatment effective.

Q: So what's the bottom line? Is there anything to clinical ecology?

A: The bottom line is that substances in the environment can indeed cause health problems. And clinical ecologists—primarily otolaryngologists (ear-nose-throat specialists), pediatricians, internists and some allergists—believe that many of the health problems people experience are caused by a sensitivity that developed because of a malfunction of the immune system. Most mainstream doctors disagree, however. And in fact, the American Academy of Allergy, Asthma and Immunology calls clinical ecology an "unproven and experimental methodology" no matter who is practicing it.

Still, there is no question that people can be adversely affected by exposure to substances in the environment. Regardless of whether you hold the traditional view of allergy or agree with the alternative view held by clinical ecologists, if you can pinpoint the substance that's causing your problem—whether it is something you are allergic to, something you are intolerant of or something to which you have some sort of sensitivity—you'd be wise to avoid it. We offer tips for avoiding some of the more common allergens in the next chapter.

8 PREVENTION

Q: Is there any way to prevent allergies from developing or to at least reduce their incidence?

A: Yes and no. As you'll recall, the standard recipe for allergy includes two key ingredients: the genetic tendency to develop an allergy and previous exposure to an allergen. Short of changing your family history or living in a vacuum 24 hours a day to limit your exposure to all of the potential allergens in the world, there is little you can do to virtually ensure that you won't develop an allergy—especially since the standard recipe is not the only recipe for allergy. After all, a small percentage of people develop allergies even if neither of their parents has them. Still, there does seem to be some evidence that careful attention to a child's diet in the first year of life can delay and reduce that child's incidence of allergy.

Q: Could you tell me more?

A: Certainly. Studies have shown that infants who have allergic parents may experience fewer allergy-related problems themselves if they are breast-fed for the first four to six months of life, particularly if their mothers avoid allergenic foods such as eggs, milk and peanuts. Breast milk is nonallergenic and provides infants with immunologic protection against infectious organisms and future food allergies. Conventional formulas made from cow's milk, on the other hand, can easily sensitize allergy-prone infants, paving the way for eczema, hay fever, asthma and gastrointestinal symptoms in years to come.

Q: How long does the protection from breast milk last?

A: A 1995 Finnish study found that it may last through adolescence. The study followed 150 infants for 17 years. One-third of the infants were breast-fed for longer than six months; one-third for between one and six months; and one-third for less than a month or not at all. Researchers found that the prevalence of allergy was highest in the group with little or no breast-feeding and lowest in the groups that were breast-fed for one month or more. By age 17, approximately 40 percent of those who were breast-fed for at least a month developed an allergic condition—eczema, food allergy or respiratory allergy—compared with 65 percent of those who either were not breast-fed at all or were breast-fed for less than one month. The incidence of substantial allergy—which researchers defined as allergy that affects more than one organ, is caused by more than one group of allergens, lasts longer than the pollen season and requires daily medication—was only 8 percent in the group breast-fed for more than six months, compared with 54 percent in the group breast-fed for less than a month or not at all.

Q: That sounds promising. But what should a parent do when her child is ready for solid food?

A: Experts recommend that solid foods be added to the diet one at a time, starting with the least allergenic foods. Most experts recommend starting with bananas and cereals such as rice and oats, then progressing to more allergenic foods. For the record, eggs, fruits, chocolate, wheat, orange juice and shellfish are among the most common causes of allergic reactions in infants and young children.

If a food allergy develops, the food should be removed from the diet.

Q: Is there anything else a parent can do to keep her child from developing allergies?

A: She might try to limit her youngster's exposure to common airborne allergens as well. (We discuss measures for reducing exposure to pollen, molds, dust and pet dander later in this chapter.) Two recent studies found that allergy-prone infants who were not exposed to food allergens and airborne allergens during their first year had significantly lower manifestations of allergies in that first year and subsequent years. Researchers speculate that avoiding allergens in infancy may raise the threshold of sensitization, lessening the chances that children will develop allergies.

Q: These measures may reduce the incidence of allergies in children, but what about people who already have allergies? Short of allergy shots or drugs, is there any way to prevent an allergy attack?

A: There certainly is. And we've discussed it throughout this book. The best way to prevent an allergy attack is to avoid the allergen or allergens that are causing it. If you can't do that, it may help to at least reduce your exposure to that allergen or allergens.

AVOIDING OUTDOOR ALLERGENS

Q: That sounds logical. But how can you avoid pollen and molds? They seem to be everywhere.

A: They are. But there are steps you can take to reduce your exposure to them. Here are some suggestions:

- Keep your windows shut to prevent pollen and mold spores from coming into your home or car. Use air-conditioning instead.
- Don't mow grass or be around freshly mowed grass. Mowing stirs up pollen and molds.
- Have someone cut down weeds near your home. Pollen concentrations are high close to the pollen source.
- Don't hang clothes or bed linens out to dry. They may collect pollen and molds.

- Avoid outdoor activities unless they're absolutely necessary.

- Know the pollen and mold seasons in your area and keep up with pollen and mold counts. While these counts may not give you an accurate picture of the pollens and molds in the air on any given day, when viewed on a year-round basis they can help you identify the beginning and end of pollen and mold seasons in your region. This will help you know when to begin taking medication.

- Shower and wash your hair after spending time outdoors on windy days when pollen and mold spore concentrations are worst. The allergens can cling to your hair.

- Avoid touching your eyes and nose. You could transfer pollen or mold spores there with your hands.

- Wash your hands often and rinse your eyes with cool water after coming indoors. This will help remove clinging pollen.

- Wear glasses or sunglasses outdoors to help keep pollen from irritating your eyes.

- Wear a filtering mask and gloves when gardening. Both medical masks and dust masks can be helpful. Dust masks are available through dealers that specialize in anti-allergy products and at many hardware stores.

- Try to stay indoors during the morning hours and when it is windy outside.

- Vacation by the beach during peak pollen season. Pollen is less common at the shore.

- Don't rake leaves. It stirs up molds.

Q: Will moving to Arizona help?

A: It's unlikely. While Arizona—and the Southwest in general—used to be relatively pollen-free, that is no longer the case. It is true that few of the region's native plants cause allergies, but a number of allergenic plants have been imported in recent years—often by allergic Easterners who wanted to bring a touch of their old homes to their new homes.

You might have more luck moving to the mountains or the seashore, as we explained in chapter 4. But even these locations are not pollen-free.

Q: I understand that. But if the pollens or molds in the region I move to are different from the ones that are causing my problems, I should be OK, shouldn't I?

A: Not necessarily. For one thing, some pollens and molds have extensive cross-reactivity, meaning you could be allergic to them simply because you're allergic to a related pollen or mold. For another, the move could expose you to new allergens to which you can become sensitized rather quickly. In other words, a move might prompt an exchange of one problem for another.

In short, unless you have other reasons for moving, you might want to avoid the hassle and expense.

AVOIDING INDOOR ALLERGENS

Q: Do you have any suggestions for avoiding indoor allergens?

A: Certainly. Let's start with dust. We'll provide you with tips for dust-proofing your entire home, but be aware that experts recommend you focus your efforts on your bedroom to give you at least one room in which dust is controlled—the one in which you spend most of your at-home hours.

- Make sure your home is cleaned regularly. But you shouldn't be the one doing the cleaning. In fact, if possible, you should leave the house during cleaning and stay away for 10 to 15 minutes afterward to give the dust time to settle. If you must do the cleaning, wear a dust mask.
- Make sure that cleanings include regular damp mopping and dusting.
- Remove dust-collecting items such as books, knickknacks and dried flower arrangements from your house.

- Replace heavy draperies or venetian blinds with washable curtains or window shades.

- Keep your bedroom and closet doors closed.

- Change or clean your air conditioner and furnace filters often.

- If your home has forced air heat, place a filter or a piece of damp cheesecloth over the inlet to reduce dust circulation. Filters are available from anti-allergy supply companies.

- Invest in an air cleaner with a HEPA (high-efficiency particulate arresting) filter. These cleaners, which can be part of your heating and cooling system or can stand alone, can be up to 99.97 percent effective in removing airborne allergens from the air.

Q: **I'd like to know more about these filters. How do they work?**

A: HEPA filters were developed during World War II to remove radioactive dust from the air. The filters are pleated to greatly increase their surface area; thus, they can eliminate very small particles—particles as small as 0.3 micron, which includes many common airborne allergens. Many HEPA filters also include charcoal prefilters to remove odors and larger particles such as hair and lint. A number of companies make and sell these air cleaners, which come in several sizes to accommodate various sizes of rooms. If you're considering purchasing an air cleaner with a HEPA filter, make sure you choose one that will adequately filter the air in the room in which you plan to use it.

Q: **What about dust mites? How can they be avoided?**

A: Remember, dust mites thrive in areas with warm temperatures and high humidity. They also like mattresses, rugs and upholstery. Altering the climate of your home and eliminating their preferred habitats will help eradicate them.

Here are some suggestions:

- Use air-conditioning to keep humidity low. This slows down mite growth during warm weather.

- Replace upholstered furniture with leather and vinyl.

- Get rid of carpeting and rugs. Hardwood floors and vinyl and linoleum floor coverings are better bets.

- If you simply must have a rug, sun it occasionally. Australian researchers recently found that placing wool rugs facedown in the direct sun for about three hours kills both dust mites and their eggs.

- Dust mites in carpeting can also be killed by applying benzyl benzoate, an acaricide sold under the brand name Acarosan.

- Break down the dust mite allergen in carpeting by applying tannic acid, a component of tea. A solution, sold under the name Allergy Control Solution, is available from anti-allergy supply stores.

- Wash your bed linens, blankets and curtains in hot water (at least 140°F) every 7 to 10 days.

- Cover mattresses and box springs with nonallergenic plastic casings.

Q: What about indoor molds? The avoidance techniques for outdoor molds don't seem to apply.

A: They do and they don't. The principle behind them is the same: You want to avoid areas that are conducive to mold growth. But the details are different. After all, no one rakes leaves or mows grass indoors. Indoor areas favorable to mold growth include the bathroom sink, the shower, the tub, the toilet, the kitchen sink, the basement, the walls and behind the refrigerator, as well as mattresses, carpet padding and upholstery.

Here are some tips for avoiding indoor molds:

- Keep the humidity level of your home below 50 percent. A dehumidifier or air conditioner may help. But because these appliances collect water, be sure to check them regularly for mold growth.

- Keep a 40-watt lightbulb lit in your basement or closet to remove darkness and deter mold growth.

- Check your house for water leaks and repair any you find.

- Remove old wallpaper and replace it with paint. Mildew-resistant paints are available.

- Don't grow plants indoors. The wet soil is conducive to mold growth.

- Replace carpeting that has gotten extensively wet or wood that has rotted as a result of water leakage.

- Keep your windows sealed as tightly as possible.

- Use chlorine bleach to clean areas in which mold is growing.

Q: **It seems like a lot of these suggestions involve making major changes—replacing furniture and carpeting and such. I'm almost afraid to ask my next question. What can be done to reduce exposure to animal allergens?**

A: If you're a pet lover, you probably won't like this answer. The most effective way to reduce exposure to animal allergens is to rid the home of the animal that produces them. For people who consider their pets part of the family, this may be easier said than done.

Short of finding another home for your pet, you may want to try keeping the pet outdoors or restricting it to one or two rooms of the house. At the very least, the pet should be kept out of the bedroom of the person who is allergic.

Here are some other suggestions that may help:

- Groom animals regularly—and do it outdoors.

- Keep caged animals such as hamsters, gerbils and guinea pigs in out-of-the-way places.

- Bathe your dog regularly.

- Consider bathing your cat. Some studies have found that this reduces cat allergens in the home, although others have disputed this finding. While the jury is still out, you may want to give it a try (if you're up to the challenge).

- If your pet favors a particular chair or sofa, cover that piece of furniture with a sheet and wash the sheet regularly.

- After playing with your pet, wash your hands or take a shower. And wash your clothes before wearing them again.
- If you are allergic to cats, have someone else change the litter box.
- Use an air cleaner to help remove pet allergens.

REDUCING ALLERGY SYMPTOMS

Q: **Could you give me any general suggestions for reducing allergy attacks and allergy symptoms?**

A: Certainly. Remember that stress, emotions, infections and diminished resistance can aggravate allergy. You'll want to do what you can to reduce stress and stay healthy. For example:

- Eat a healthy, well-balanced diet.
- Get adequate sleep.
- Exercise.
- Try deep breathing exercises or other relaxation techniques.

Q: **That's certainly logical advice. Are there any other things I can do?**

A: Yes. Allergies—particularly respiratory allergies—can also be aggravated by cigarette smoke, perfumes, chemicals and other inhaled irritants. If possible, try to avoid these offending substances. It won't make your allergies disappear, but it might lessen the severity of your symptoms.

If these environmental changes don't bring your allergies under control, you may wish to couple them with medication and/or immunotherapy. We discuss these medical approaches to allergy control in the next two chapters.

9 MEDICAL MANAGEMENT

Q: I know allergies can't be cured, but you said they can often be controlled. How?

A: As we've said throughout this book, the most effective way to control allergic disease—regardless of the form it takes—is to avoid the allergen or allergens that are causing it. If you're allergic to a food, you shouldn't eat it. If you're allergic to a drug, you shouldn't take it—or you should at least discuss your allergy with your doctor. If you're allergic to cats or dogs, you shouldn't keep them as pets. But sometimes it's not so simple. For example, it can be hard to avoid a food if you are unaware that it is an ingredient of another food—that it's hidden. Likewise, it can be hard to avoid even minimal exposure to pollen and molds when you are outdoors at certain times of the year. In these cases—when you can't avoid the allergen or sufficiently reduce your exposure to it—a variety of medical treatments can be used to bring allergy under control.

Q: What do you mean, under control?

A: Medical treatments can be used to alleviate symptoms or to lessen their severity. They can also be used to prevent allergy attacks and, in the case of immunotherapy (allergy shots), to lessen a person's sensitivity to an allergen. Decreased sensitivity would, of course, both reduce the number of allergy attacks the person experiences and lessen the severity of her symptoms. In other words, medical treatments can make it possible for most people with allergies to lead normal lives.

Q: That's certainly promising! I'd like to know more. What types of medical treatments are there?

A: There are two types of medical treatments for allergies: drugs and immunotherapy. We discuss immunotherapy in chapter 10. Drugs used to treat allergies include antihistamines, **decongestants**, antihistamine-decongestant combinations, anti-inflammatory drugs and epinephrine. People with allergic asthma may also require other medications—specifically **broncho-dilators** and **mucokinetic drugs**.

ANTIHISTAMINES

Q: You've already mentioned antihistamines, and I've heard the term before. Aren't they what people take to treat their colds?

A: A number of cold medications do indeed contain antihistamines, and if you think about the similarities between cold symptoms and the symptoms of allergic rhinitis, you'll probably see why. Antihistamines counteract the symptoms of rhinitis—the inflammation of the nose common to both colds and allergies. As a result, they are used to treat both conditions. But while antihistamines may relieve the itchy, runny nose of rhinitis, they are also effective in countering many of histamine's other effects. They literally work against histamine.

Q: I know we've talked about histamine before, but could you refresh my memory? What is it, and what does it do?

A: Histamine is a chemical mediator contained in mast cells and basophils. When it is released into the body, it makes blood vessels widen and release fluid, resulting in swelling. It also irritates nerve endings, causing itching.

In allergy, histamine is released only after an allergen enters the body and meets up with an immunoglobulin E antibody attached to a mast cell or a basophil. Mast cells, as you'll recall, are located in the skin, nose, lungs and gastrointestinal tract, while basophils circulate through the bloodstream. Depending on the location of these cells, the release of histamine can cause a variety of allergic symptoms. If histamine is released in nasal passages, for example, the nose can become inflamed, swollen and itchy. Likewise, if it is released in the eyes, the eyes can become itchy and swollen and may start to water. Released in the skin, histamine can cause the wheals and itching of hives; in the lungs, it can provoke asthma; and in the gastrointestinal tract, it can cause cramps and the increased secretion of fluids. And if histamine is released throughout the entire body, it can trigger anaphylaxis.

Q: **So a drug that counteracts histamine's effects can relieve a variety of allergy symptoms, right?**

A: Right. Antihistamines are commonly used to treat the symptoms of allergic rhinitis, allergic conjunctivitis and hives. They are also used in conjunction with other medications to treat anaphylaxis and, occasionally, asthma.

Q: **How do antihistamines work?**

A: Before we can explain the mechanism of antihistamines, you need to know a little more about the mechanism of histamine. We've told you what histamine is and what it does, but you need to know what happens between the time it is released from mast cells and basophils and the time it begins to dilate blood vessels and irritate nerve endings. When histamine is released, it connects with **receptors** on the surface of cells throughout the body. It is only after this connection is made that histamine begins to exert its effects.

Antihistamines work by beating histamine to the punch. Antihistamines have a molecular structure similar to histamine and, therefore, can connect with histamine receptors. If antihistamines reach the receptors first, they leave histamine with no place to go. Histamine that cannot connect with histamine receptors cannot start the chain of events that completes its part of an allergic reaction. In other words, antihistamines interrupt the allergic reaction that begins when allergen and IgE antibody meet, triggering histamine's release.

Q: I think I understand, but one thing has me confused. You said that antihistamines work by beating histamine to the punch. Wouldn't a person have to take an antihistamine before her allergic reaction begins in order for the drug to be effective?

A: Yes and no. Antihistamines are indeed most effective if they are taken before allergy symptoms appear. This is because allergy symptoms are in large part the result of histamine action, and antihistamines can do nothing to relieve the effects of the histamine that has already begun to act on the body. But remember, there's more to an allergic reaction than the initial release of histamine from mast cells. As we explained in chapter 2, mediators released from the mast cells spark the production of eosinophils. These cells in turn release chemicals that trigger basophils to release histamine into the blood. And in some people, a second, late-phase reaction occurs. Thus, antihistamines taken during the early stages of an allergic reaction may still be effective, preventing existing symptoms from worsening or additional symptoms from developing. And depending on which antihistamine is used, the drug can continue to work in the body for hours.

Antihistamines work best, however, if you anticipate your need for them and take them before you are exposed to an allergen.

Q: How can I anticipate my need for them?

A: That depends on what's causing your problem. If mold or pollen is your problem, for example, you need to pay attention to mold counts or pollen counts. If you know that the tree you're allergic to usually pollinates in March, watch the calendar. And if you're allergic to dog dander, anticipate problems before you visit that new neighbor who's constantly outside whistling for Rover and Fido.

Q: All of those allergens can cause allergic rhinitis. Is that what antihistamines are generally used to treat?

A: Antihistamines are highly effective in controlling the nasal itching, runny nose and sneezing of allergic rhinitis and, consequently, are among the drugs of choice for treating this most common form of allergic disease. Because they are less effective in treating nasal congestion, however, they are often taken in conjunction with decongestants. We talk more about decongestants and antihistamine-decongestant combinations later in this chapter.

Antihistamines are also among the primary treatments for allergic conjunctivitis and for hives. They relieve itching, redness and tearing of the eyes; they relieve the itching of hives; and they reduce the size, number and duration of wheals. In fact, many people with chronic hives are treated solely with a combination of two types of antihistamines.

Q: Two types?

A: Yes. We already said that antihistamines work by connecting with histamine receptors. Well, there are several distinct types of histamine receptors, two of which play roles in allergy. Consequently, two distinct types of antihistamines are used to treat allergic conditions.

The first is the **H_1 antihistamines**, which compete with histamine to connect with H_1 receptors located throughout the body. This is the type of antihistamine most commonly used to treat allergy. The second type, the **H_2 antihistamines**, compete with histamine to connect with H_2 receptors, which are most common in the lining of the stomach. These H_2 blockers, which are often used to treat stomach problems, are occasionally used in conjunction with H_1 antihistamines to treat hives.

Q: Why?

A: Because when histamine works through both H_1 and H_2 receptors, it reduces blood pressure and causes flushing—symptoms that are present in some people with chronic hives.

H₁ Antihistamines

Q: I'd like to know more about both of these drugs, starting with the H_1 antihistamines. What forms do they come in? Are they available over the counter? Do they have any side effects?

A: Slow down. Let's tackle one question at a time. H_1 antihistamines come in several forms. There are topical forms—nasal sprays, eyedrops and skin creams and sprays—and there are oral forms—capsules, tablets and liquids.

The topical forms, obviously, are used specifically to counter symptoms in the areas in which they're applied. Nasal sprays are used to relieve nasal itching and sneezing; eyedrops are used to relieve itching and redness in the eyes; and topical creams and sprays are used to relieve the itching and swelling of allergic rashes. The oral forms are used to treat a wide variety of allergy symptoms throughout the body.

Q: Are both topical and oral H_1 antihistamines available over the counter?

A: Yes. In fact, the majority of topical H_1 antihistamines are available without a prescription.

Q: Could you give me some examples of topical H_1 antihistamines available over the counter?

A: Certainly. These include but are not limited to:

Nasal sprays
- pyrilamine (4-Way Fast Acting Nasal Spray)
- pheniramine (Dristan Nasal Spray)

Eyedrops
- pheniramine (Opcon-A, OcuHist, Naphcon-A)

Topical creams and sprays
- diphenhydramine (Benadryl, Dermarest)

Q: What about the oral H_1 antihistamines? Could you give me some examples of them?

A: Of course. H_1 antihistamines available with a prescription include:
- pyrilamine (Atrohist, R-Tannate, Rynatan, Triotann)
- tripelennamine (PBZ)
- clemastine (Tavist)
- diphenhydramine (Benadryl)
- brompheniramine (Bromfed)
- hydroxyzine (Atarax)
- cyproheptadine (Periactin)
- promethazine (Phenergan)

These drugs may be included in other prescription drug preparations. In addition, there are prescription-strength versions of several H_1 antihistamines that are available without a prescription.

Q: Which H_1 antihistamines are available without a prescription?

A: Nonprescription H_1 antihistamines—many of which are sold in combination with decongestants—are available in a variety of store, generic and national brands. Here are the generic names of these antihistamines, followed by some examples of national brands:
- diphenhydramine (Benadryl)
- clemastine (Tavist-1)
- brompheniramine (Dimetapp Allergy)
- chlorpheniramine (Efidac 24, Chlor-Trimeton Allergy; also found in Comtrex, Contac Allergy Timed-Release, Coricidin and Tylenol Allergy Sinus Medication)
- pyrilamine (found in Triaminic products)
- doxylamine (found in Contac Nighttime Cold Medicine and Vicks Nyquil)

- dexbrompheniramine (found in Drixoral products and Sinutab Allergy Formula)
- triprolidine (found in Actifed products)

These antihistamines are also found in numerous generic- and store-brand cold and allergy medications.

Q: **Hey, I've heard of a lot of those! I've even taken a few of them when I've had colds. But if I remember correctly, they made me sleepy. Is that possible?**

A: Yes. In fact, drowsiness is the most common side effect of many H_1 antihistamines, including those available without a prescription. Many H_1 antihistamines also diminish alertness, slow reaction time and impair thinking—symptoms that, like drowsiness, result from the drugs' effects on the central nervous system.

Q: **Do H_1 antihistamines have any other side effects?**

A: Yes. Other side effects can include upset stomach, increased appetite, dry mouth, nervousness, fatigue, blurred vision, urinary retention, heart palpitations, irregular heartbeat and impotence. Fortunately, however, these side effects are far less common than drowsiness. And with continued use of these drugs, some people develop a tolerance for drowsiness and other central nervous system side effects. They simply stop experiencing them.

Q: **Aren't there H_1 antihistamines that don't make a person sleepy?**

A: Yes. Several of the newer H_1 antihistamines, commonly referred to as second-generation antihistamines, are relatively nonsedating. In fact, these drugs have very few adverse effects on the central nervous system. However, none of these nonsedating, second-generation antihistamines is currently available without a prescription.

Q: What are the names of these drugs?

A: The nonsedating antihistamines are:

- terfenadine (Seldane)
- astemizole (Hismanal)
- loratadine (Claritin)
- cetirizine (Zyrtec)
- fexofenadine hydrochloride (Allegra)

Q: Didn't I hear somewhere that Seldane is dangerous?

A: While Seldane generally poses few problems on its own if it is taken at recommended doses, it may cause problems when it is taken in conjunction with certain other drugs or when it is taken in excessive amounts. Seldane, the first nonsedating antihistamine approved for use in the United States, has been known to cause fatal or near-fatal heartbeat abnormalities and heart attacks when it is taken in excess or when it is taken in conjunction with the antibiotics erythromycin, clarithromycin and troleandomycin or with the antifungal drugs ketoconazole and itraconazole. In 1992, the Food and Drug Administration mandated that Seldane carry a warning on its label indicating that it should not be used in conjunction with those drugs. Similar problems have been reported for Hismanal, and a similar warning appears on the package.

None of the other three nonsedating antihistamines—Claritin, Zyrtec and Allegra—poses similar problems.

Q: So which are better for treating allergies—the newer, nonsedating antihistamines or the older ones that can make a person sleepy?

A: That depends on the person's needs. First-generation and second-generation H_1 antihistamines are both effective in treating allergy. For people for whom drowsiness does not pose a problem—perhaps they take the drug at night before bed—first-generation antihistamines may be the best bet. They are less expensive than their newer counterparts, and many of them can be obtained over the counter. For people who must remain alert, however, the newer, nonsedating antihistamines may be a better choice.

H_2 Antihistamines

Q: What about the other kind of antihistamines you mentioned—the ones that work on the H_2 receptors?

A: In recent years, H_2 antihistamines have been used in conjunction with H_1 antihistamines to treat hives. H_2 antihistamines work by blocking histamine from H_2 receptors, which are prevalent in the lining of the stomach. These drugs— which include cimetidine (Tagamet), ranitidine hydrochloride (Zantac) and famotidine (Pepcid)—are primarily used to treat stomach and duodenal ulcers and to relieve the effects of heart-burn. Several of these drugs have recently become available over the counter.

Q: Do they have any side effects?

A: Side effects are rare. On occasion, people taking H_2 antihistamines report headaches and confusion; less commonly, they report constipation, liver dysfunction, rashes and loss of interest in sex.

Q: Are these antihistamines ever used by themselves in the treatment of allergy?

A: Not at the present time.

Q: Why is that?

A: Because while H_2 receptors may work with H_1 receptors in triggering some allergy symptoms, when they act alone they simply increase the secretion of gastric acid in the stomach. Most allergy symptoms result from histamine's connection with H_1 receptors. Thus, it is the H_1 antihistamines that are the mainstays of allergy management.

DECONGESTANTS

Q: You said that antihistamines are often used in conjunction with decongestants. What are decongestants?

A: Decongestants are drugs that reduce swelling. When they reduce swelling in the nasal passages, they reduce congestion—hence the name decongestant.

Q: How do decongestants reduce swelling?

A: As you'll recall, when histamine is released, it causes blood vessels to dilate, which enables fluid from those blood vessels to leak into the surrounding tissues. This causes swelling. When that swelling occurs in the lining of the nose, it reduces the size of the passages through which air flows and creates a congested, stuffed-up feeling.

Decongestants make those swollen blood vessels constrict, stopping the leakage of fluid into the tissues and allowing the tissues to shrink back to their normal size. In the nose, this opens up the nasal passages, giving more room for air to pass.

Q: What forms do decongestants come in?

A: There are two general types: topical decongestants, which are sprayed or dropped directly into the nose, and systemic decongestants, which are taken orally and come in liquids, capsules and tablets.

Topical Decongestants

Q: I'd like to know about both types, starting with the topical drugs. What are they used for?

A: Topical decongestants are used to provide quick, temporary relief from nasal congestion caused by a cold or allergy. The relief is quick—within minutes—because the drug is delivered directly to the area on which it will work. The relief is temporary, however, because topical decongestants should not be used for more than three to five days or more frequently than recommended.

Q: Why is that?

A: Because continued use of a topical decongestant shortens the drug's effectiveness and leads to a rebound reaction— a more severe form of congestion—after the drug is discontinued. This is called **rhinitis medicamentosa**. And it's a very good reason to follow directions on the label carefully.

Q: It certainly is. Are there any other side effects of topical decongestants?

A: Yes. Fortunately, these side effects are generally limited to the nose. They include burning, stinging and the sensation of dryness.

Q: Are topical decongestants available over the counter?

A: Yes. While a few topical decongestants are available only by prescription, a large number are available over the counter. These include:

- phenylephrine (Dristan Nasal Spray, Neo-Synephrine, Duration, Sinex, 4-Way Fast Acting Nasal Spray)
- oxymetazoline (Afrin, Coricidin, Duration, Nostrilla, 4-Way Long Acting Nasal Spray)
- naphazoline (4-Way Fast Acting Nasal Spray)
- xylometazoline (Otrivin)

Systemic Decongestants

Q: What about the systemic decongestants? When are they used?

A: Systemic decongestants, like topical decongestants, are used to relieve nasal congestion caused by colds and allergies. Unlike topical decongestants, however, they can be used for extended periods of time. This is because they rarely cause rebound nasal congestion.

Q: Do systemic decongestants have any side effects?

A: They do. Because they have a stimulant effect, they have been known to make people jumpy and irritable, increase heartbeat, prompt headaches, cause insomnia and raise blood pressure. Because of these side effects, people with high blood pressure or heart disease should talk with their doctors before using systemic decongestants.

Q: Are systemic decongestants available without a prescription?

A: They are. A variety of forms and dosages of the two major decongestants—pseudoephedrine and phenylpropanolamine—are available over the counter. Common brands of pseudoephedrine include:

- Sudafed
- Dimetapp (Decongestant)
- Efidac 24 (Decongestant)
- Actifed Sinus Daytime
- Sine-Aid
- Robitussin Severe Congestion

Common brands of phenylpropanolamine include:
- Vicks Dayquil
- Contac 12-Hour Cold

Both pseudoephedrine and phenylpropanolamine are also found in a host of generic- and store-brand products as well as in products that also include antihistamines.

ANTIHISTAMINE-DECONGESTANT COMBINATIONS

Q: What is the point of combining a decongestant with an antihistamine?

A: Antihistamines are effective in relieving the sneezing, the itchy, runny nose and the itchy, watery eyes of allergic rhinitis. But because they do not cause blood vessels that have been dilated by histamine to constrict, they are not effective at relieving nasal congestion. Decongestants, on the other hand, are effective at relieving nasal congestion but do nothing for the other symptoms of allergic rhinitis. As a result, many people with allergic rhinitis need both antihistamines and decongestants to address all of their symptoms; thus, a variety of products on the market contain both types of drugs.

Q: Are these combinations available over the counter?

A: Yes. Antihistamine-decongestant combinations are available both with and without a prescription. They vary according to the actual drugs used in the combination and the doses of each individual drug. Combination products sold over the counter generally include one of four antihistamines—brompheniramine, chlorpheniramine, dexbrompheniramine or triprolidine—and one of two decongestants—pseudoephedrine or phenylpropanolamine. Doses vary according to the combination of drugs used and how the drugs are formulated. Some combination drugs must be taken every 4 to 6 hours; others must be taken less frequently—say, every 12 or every 24 hours.

Q: What about the prescription combinations? Do they use the same drugs?

A: Some do, some don't. Atrohist, for example, combines chlorpheniramine with pseudoephedrine, while Claritin-D and Seldane-D combine prescription, nonsedating antihistamines with pseudoephedrine.

Prescription combinations may include more than one decongestant, more than one antihistamine or drugs designed to alleviate other symptoms such as coughing or pain. Or they may simply include higher doses of drugs used in over-the-counter preparations.

Q: Those combination products sound convenient. But couldn't I achieve the same effect by taking two different drugs, one an antihistamine and one a decongestant?

A: Yes. And in fact, many people do just that. If your symptoms vary, you may want to vary your treatment accordingly. If your only symptom is nasal stuffiness, for example, you should take a decongestant and leave it at that. Likewise, if your nose is runny or itchy but you do not feel congested, you should choose an antihistamine. And if you occasionally experience a combination of symptoms, you may want to take both an antihistamine and a decongestant. Whether to take separate medications or a combination medication is strictly a matter of choice.

ANTI-INFLAMMATORY DRUGS

Q: At the beginning of this chapter, you mentioned anti-inflammatory drugs. What are they, and what role do they play in managing allergy?

A: Anti-inflammatory drugs, as their name implies, are drugs that counter inflammation.

You'll recall from chapter 2 that allergic reactions cause inflammation. This occurs when histamine and other mediators dilate blood vessels and make them more permeable as well as stimulate nerve endings. At the same time, the white blood cells known as neutrophils release enzymes and other chemicals to attack the allergen, which adds to the inflammation. Anti-inflammatory drugs reduce or prevent the pain, swelling, redness and heat—the inflammation—caused by allergic reactions.

Q: What types of allergies are anti-inflammatory drugs used to treat?

A: Anti-inflammatory drugs are used to treat both respiratory allergies (allergic rhinitis and asthma) and skin allergies (hives and contact dermatitis). They are also used to treat ocular, or eye, allergies. The two major types of anti-inflammatory drugs used to treat allergy are the **mast-cell stabilizers** and the corticosteroids.

Mast-Cell Stabilizers

Q: I know what a mast cell is, but what is a mast-cell stabilizer?

A: A mast-cell stabilizer is a drug that stabilizes mast cells, preventing them from releasing histamine and other mediators. As you might imagine, if mast cells cannot release

histamine and other mediators, allergy symptoms do not occur.
The allergic reaction is literally stopped before it begins. Thus,
mast-cell stabilizers, unlike antihistamines and decongestants, have
a **prophylactic**—meaning preventive—action. The oldest and
most well known mast-cell stabilizer is **cromolyn sodium**.

Q: How is cromolyn sodium used?

A: Cromolyn sodium is usually applied directly to the
mast cells that would normally be affected by allergy. It
comes in three forms: a nasal spray (for allergic rhinitis), eyedrops
(for allergic conjunctivitis) and a product that can be inhaled
(for asthma).

Q: Could you tell me more about the nasal spray?

A: Certainly. Cromolyn sodium nasal spray (Nasalcrom),
which is available only by prescription, is used to prevent
the symptoms of allergic rhinitis. As such, it is most effective if
treatment begins before allergy season starts and continues
throughout the season or, in the case of perennial allergic rhinitis,
if it is used regularly.

Cromolyn sodium can also be used on an as-needed basis to
reduce symptoms from exposure to specific, known allergens.
If, for example, you are allergic to cats and know you are going
to come in contact with one, you might want to use the nasal
spray beforehand.

Q: Are there any side effects?

A: The most common side effect of cromolyn sodium nasal
spray is sneezing. Other side effects include burning and
stinging in the nose, a bad taste in the mouth, nasal bleeding
and increased postnasal drip.

Q: What about the eyedrops?

A: Cromolyn sodium eye drops, sold under the brand name Crolom and also available only by prescription, are used to alleviate itching, tearing and discomfort of the eyes. The major side effect is burning.

Q: And the asthma medication?

A: The form of cromolyn sodium used to treat asthma, sold under the brand name Intal, can be inhaled from a metered-dose inhaler (a device that houses a small aerosol cannister filled with medication), as a nebulized liquid (a liquid dispensed as a fine mist) or by means of a powder-filled capsule placed in a Spinhaler, a small device that punctures the capsule and propels the powder into the lungs. A new form of cromolyn sodium, Gastrocom, is a powder that can be dissolved in water and taken as a drink.

Cromolyn sodium can be either inhaled 15 minutes before exercise or exposure to allergens or taken regularly as part of an asthma maintenance program. It generally takes at least a month of regular use to determine whether cromolyn sodium is effective; cromolyn sodium doesn't work for every asthmatic person.

Q: Does the form of cromolyn sodium used to treat asthma have any side effects?

A: The side effects are very few. The most common is wheezing or coughing after inhalation of the powder. Throat irritation, dry mouth, nasal congestion, nasal bleeding and a bad taste in the mouth have occasionally been reported.

Q: Are any drugs similar to cromolyn sodium used to treat allergy?

A: Yes. Since the early 1990s, two similar drugs have become available to treat allergic conjunctivitis.

Lodoxamide (Alomide), like cromolyn sodium, is a mast-cell stabilizer, while ketorolac tromethamine (Acular) works by inhibiting the creation of prostaglandins, chemical mediators that, like histamine, play a role in allergic reactions. The primary side effects of both drugs are stinging and burning.

There is also a new anti-inflammatory drug for asthma, nedocromil sodium (Tilade), which appears to prohibit the release of mediators from a variety of different kinds of cells.

Corticosteroids

Q: **What about the other drugs you mentioned— the corticosteroids? What are they used to treat?**

A: Corticosteroids, commonly called steroids, are used to treat both respiratory and skin allergies. Like antihistamines and decongestants, they come in both topical and systemic forms.

Q: **Aren't steroids dangerous?**

A: There are many types of steroids, and some of them are indeed dangerous. But the corticosteroids used to treat allergy and asthma are completely different from the anabolic steroids sometimes used by weight lifters and other athletes interested in building muscle mass.

Topical corticosteroids are relatively safe; very little gets into the bloodstream to cause side effects. Systemic corticosteroids do pose some problems, however. We'll address this issue shortly.

Topical

Q: **In the meantime, could you tell me more about the topical corticosteroids? Which allergies are they used to treat?**

A: Topical corticosteroids are used to treat allergic rhinitis, asthma, allergic contact dermatitis and eczema. The form in which they are used varies according to the allergy they are used to treat: nasal sprays and inhalers for respiratory allergies, creams and ointments for skin allergies.

Q: **What do the nasal sprays do?**

A: More potent than antihistamines, decongestants and mast-cell stabilizers, corticosteroid nasal sprays decrease swelling, blood vessel dilation and inflammation in the nose. They do this by blocking the formation and release of histamine and other mediators, by reducing the number of inflammatory cells present in the nasal mucosa and by decreasing the sensitivity of the nerves that cause sneezing.

Q: **Are these effects immediate?**

A: No. It takes from one to three weeks to achieve the maximum benefit from a spray, which must be used regularly from one to four times a day, depending on the drug. The sprays are most effective in treating seasonal allergic rhinitis when treatment begins prior to the allergy season and is continued through until the end of the season.

Q: **Are nasal corticosteroids available over the counter?**

A: These drugs—which include beclomethasone (Beconase, Vancenase), triamcinolone (Nasacort) and the newcomers fluticasone (Flonase) and budesonide (Rhinocort)—are currently available only by prescription.

Some of the same drugs are also available via inhalers for the treatment of asthma.

Q: What effect do these drugs have on asthma?

A: Inhaled steroids have the same anti-inflammatory effects as steroid nasal sprays, but they reduce inflammation in the lungs, not in the nose.

Q: Do steroid sprays and inhalers have any side effects?

A: The sprays can cause nasal irritation, nosebleeds, nasal congestion and headaches. Inhaled steroids can cause a fungal infection of the mouth known as thrush, but this can be prevented by rinsing the mouth after each inhalation.

Q: What about corticosteroid creams and ointments? How do they work?

A: Topical steroid creams and ointments also work by relieving inflammation—in this instance, inflamed skin. They are effective treatments for poison ivy and other forms of allergic contact dermatitis as well as for acute flare-ups of eczema. They come in a variety of potencies.

Q: Are any of these creams and ointments available without a prescription?

A: Yes. A number of low-potency corticosteroid creams and ointments are available over the counter; high-potency drugs are available with a prescription. The over-the-counter preparations, most of which feature hydrocortisone as their major ingredient, are often effective in bringing poison ivy and other outbreaks of contact dermatitis under control when used for one to two weeks. Severe cases may require more potent prescription medications, however.

Q: What about eczema?

A: Topical steroid creams and ointments are often used to treat acute flare-ups of atopic dermatitis. Some people with severe eczema may need to use the products continually, but this is not generally recommended.

Q: Why is that?

A: There are several reasons. While topical steroid creams are not taken directly into the bloodstream, they are absorbed through the skin. Thus, continued or widespread use may cause systemic side effects. In addition, prolonged use of high-potency topical steroids can cause the skin to thin. And long-term application around the eyes or eyelids can lead to glaucoma or cataracts (a clouding of the lens of the eye that obstructs vision).

Fortunately, the side effects of topical steroid creams and ointments are usually minimal. They can include itching, dryness and loss of skin color.

Systemic

Q: I take it the side effects of the systemic corticosteroids are not so minimal?

A: You're right. Systemic corticosteroids, which can be taken orally or injected, may cause serious side effects, which is why they are available only by prescription. The side effects occur because steroids can suppress the body's normal production of adrenal hormones, which are vital to the function of many organs in the body. This occurs primarily with long-term use.

Q: What are the side effects of long-term use?

A: They include high blood pressure, diabetes, the development of cataracts and glaucoma, ulcers, osteoporosis (loss of bone mass) and an impaired immune system.

Q: Are there any side effects when the drugs are used only for a short time?

A: Yes. They include increased appetite, fluid retention, weight gain, muscle weakness, acne, high blood pressure and moodiness.

Q: Whew! Sounds like these drugs are more trouble than they're worth. Why are they even used?

A: Because they can be extremely effective in relieving allergy symptoms when other drugs cannot. In fact, the failure of other drugs to relieve symptoms is the major indication for prescribing systemic corticosteroids for allergy.

Q: Which allergy symptoms can they help alleviate?

A: Systemic corticosteroids such as prednisone (Deltasone, Prednicen-M, Sterapred), methylprednisolone (Medrol), dexamethasone (Decadron) and triamcinolone (Aristocort) can clear up severe cases of hives and stubborn cases of allergic contact dermatitis. They can also provide dramatic relief from severe flare-ups of asthma and allergic rhinitis. In most instances, the drugs are taken only for a short time.

Q: How long?

A: That depends, of course, on the nature of the problem and on the person's response to the drugs. In general, however, the drugs are prescribed for anywhere from several days to two to three weeks. The dose is often tapered off gradually.

Q: Why is that?

A: You'll recall that systemic corticosteroids suppress the body's production of adrenal hormones. If the drugs are stopped abruptly, the body may not have the hormones it needs. This can send the body into shock. If you are taking systemic corticosteroids, never discontinue them without a doctor's orders.

Q: Are systemic steroids ever prescribed for long-term use?

A: Yes. Systemic steroids are prescribed on a long-term basis for people with severe chronic asthma and, on occasion, for people with severe chronic hives. This long-term therapy may require daily or alternate-day doses. Alternate-day doses minimize the hormone suppression caused by the drugs. Ultimately, however, the goal is to wean the person from the steroids altogether, if possible.

EPINEPHRINE

Q: Isn't the drug used to treat anaphylaxis also a hormonelike drug?

A: Yes. Epinephrine is a synthetic form of a naturally occurring hormone that stimulates the nervous system and the heart.

Q: Does it pose the same problems as corticosteroids?

A: No. Epinephrine is not used for long periods of time. Therefore, it has no long-lasting side effects.

Q: How does epinephrine work?

A: Epinephrine is injected into the body of a person experiencing anaphylaxis, an acute asthma attack or, on occasion, severe acute hives. It constricts the blood vessels, raises lowered blood pressure, increases the heart rate and relaxes smooth muscles in the airways, opening closed respiratory passages.

Q: You said epinephrine is injected. By whom?

A: That depends. People who have experienced anaphylactic symptoms in the past—people allergic to peanuts or insect venom, for example—are often prescribed kits with injectable epinephrine to use in case of emergency. These kits, sold under the brand names EpiPen and EpiPen Jr., contain a premeasured amount of epinephrine in an injector that's designed so that the person experiencing symptoms can inject the drug into his thigh. In other cases—cases in which the person is unaware of an allergy or does not have an emergency kit—the injection is given by emergency medical personnel after the person experiencing problems has sought treatment.

Q: Are any other drugs used to treat anaphylaxis?

A: Epinephrine is the primary treatment. In some instances, however, antihistamines, corticosteroids and, occasionally, bronchodilators may be used in conjunction with epinephrine.

ASTHMA MEDICATIONS

Q: What are bronchodilators?

A: Bronchodilators are drugs that open airways by relaxing constricted muscles. They are used to counteract the bronchospasms of asthma. Epinephrine itself can be used as a bronchodilator, although it is rarely used in day-to-day asthma management.

Q: What bronchodilators are used to manage asthma?

A: Three types of bronchodilators are used to manage asthma: sympathomimetics, xanthines and anti-cholinergics. The most commonly used sympathomimetic drugs are beta-adrenergic agonists (also called beta-adrenergic stimulants, beta-agonists or beta-2 agonists), which include albuterol (Proventil, Ventolin), bitolterol (Tornalate), pirbuterol (Maxair), salmeterol (Serevent), metaproterenol (Alupent) and terbutaline (Brethaire, Brethine, Bricanyl). These drugs are used either on an as-needed basis to treat asthma symptoms and prevent exercise-induced asthma attacks or on a daily basis as part of a plan to control chronic asthma.

Q: What about the other types of bronchodilators?

A: The xanthines, which include theophylline (Aerolate, Quibron, Respbid, Slo-bid, Theo-Dur) and aminophylline (available only in combination with other drugs), are used to relax bronchial muscles and are prescribed in short-acting, intermediate-acting and long-acting forms. The anticholinergics, which include atropine (available only in combination with other drugs) and **ipratropium bromide** (Atrovent), open airways and block the production of chemicals that cause bronchospasms.

Medications Used to Treat Allergy Symptoms

Symptom	Medication(s)
Respiratory Allergies	
Allergic rhinitis	
Nasal congestion	Decongestants (oral and topical)
Itchy, runny nose	Antihistamines, mast-cell stabilizers, topical corticosteroids
Itchy, watery eyes	Antihistamines, mast-cell stabilizers
Nasal congestion; itchy, runny nose; and itchy, watery eyes	Antihistamine-decongestant combinations, mast-cell stabilizers, topical corticosteroids
Asthma	Antihistamines, bronchodilators, mast-cell stabilizers, mucokinetic drugs, systemic corticosteroids, topical corticosteroids
Skin Allergies	
Atopic dermatitis	Antihistamines (to control itching), topical corticosteroids
Contact dermatitis	Antihistamines, systemic corticosteroids, topical corticosteroids
Hives	Antihistamines, epinephrine, systemic corticosteroids
Systemic Reactions	
Anaphylaxis	Antihistamines, bronchodilators, epinephrine, systemic corticosteroids

Q: Didn't you say that people with asthma may also require another type of drug?

A: Yes. People with asthma may also require mucokinetic drugs, which help clear mucus from the lungs. Also known as expectorants, these drugs are common ingredients in a number of prescription and over-the-counter cough syrups. One example of this type of drug is guaifenesin, which is a component of prescription drugs such as Deconsal, GuaiMAX-D and Humibid and of over-the-counter medications such as Robitussin DM, Comtrex Deep Chest Cold and Vicks Dayquil, among others. These drugs enable asthmatic people to cough up more mucus.

For more information about asthma medications, we refer you to our book *Asthma: Questions You Have ... Answers You Need.*

ON THE HORIZON

Q: Are there any other medications that may become a part of allergy management in the future?

A: Yes. A new form of the bronchodilator ipratropium bromide came on the market in 1996. This nasal spray, also marketed under the name Atrovent, is indicated for the relief of runny nose associated with allergic rhinitis and the common cold. Although the drug is not effective in treating sneezing, itching, watery eyes, congestion or postnasal drip, it may benefit people whose runny noses are not helped by antihistamines alone.

People with asthma may benefit from a new class of drugs, **leukotriene receptor antagonists**. The first of these drugs, zafirlukast (Accolate), received approval from the Food and Drug Administration in late 1996. These drugs compete with leukotrienes, chemical mediators that contribute to both asthma and allergy symptoms, to reach leukotriene receptors in much the same way that antihistamines compete with histamine for histamine receptors.

And pharmaceutical researchers are hard at work trying to develop drugs that address other stages of the allergic reaction.

Q: Such as?

A: Some pharmaceutical companies are attempting to create genetically engineered antibodies that will bind with the IgE antibody before it connects with a mast cell. As you'll recall, once an IgE antibody connects with a mast cell, it stays there. And when it connects with its allergen, it causes the mast cell to release histamine and other mediators.

Yet another approach is to prevent the production of the IgE antibody itself. One pharmaceutical company is working to create a new form of interleukin that could attach itself to B cells, leaving the type of interleukin that stimulates B cells to produce IgE with no place to go.

Q: Anything else?

A: In addition to looking for new ways to stop allergic reactions in their tracks, pharmaceutical companies are working to improve tried-and-true treatments. New antihistamines and corticosteroid nasal sprays are being developed and approved at a rapid pace, and pharmaceutical companies are working to develop a nasal form of immunotherapy that could ultimately replace allergy shots. As yet, however, there is no cure for allergy. At this point, immunotherapy is the closest we can get.

10 IMMUNOTHERAPY

Q: You said immunotherapy is the closest thing to a cure for allergy. In what way?

A: The goal of immunotherapy, or allergy shots, is to desensitize a person to an allergen to which he is sensitized. When immunotherapy is successful, a person's sensitivity to an allergen decreases and, in some cases, disappears. Thus, it decreases both the frequency and the severity of allergy symptoms. It can also reduce a person's need for medication.

Approximately 85 percent of patients with allergic rhinitis obtain long-lasting symptom relief with immunotherapy. Sixty percent of these people continue to benefit from the shots—with reduced need for medication—after immunotherapy is discontinued.

Q: That sounds promising. What about other allergic conditions? What does immunotherapy do for them?

A: Immunotherapy is generally used only in the management of allergic rhinitis and allergic asthma. Food allergies, which often cause hives, and hives caused by other allergies simply do not respond well to immunotherapy. And while eczema is occasionally helped by allergy shots, this relief generally occurs only when eczema is accompanied by allergic rhinitis, asthma or both conditions.

Q: What's the theory behind immunotherapy?

A: Immunotherapy, or desensitization therapy, is based on the theory that if the body is gradually exposed to small doses of an allergen, the body may in time become desensitized to that allergen, so it will no longer trigger an allergic reaction.

Q: What does immunotherapy involve?

A: Immunotherapy involves a series of injections of allergen extract or extracts, commonly referred to as allergy shots. These extracts, like those used in allergy skin tests, contain the specific protein or proteins that cause your allergic reaction.

Q: What do these extracts do?

A: The extracts stimulate the production of immunoglobulin G antibodies specific to the allergens in the injection solution. Later, when you are exposed to the actual allergens, these IgG antibodies bind with those allergens. This prevents the allergens from binding with the immunoglobulin E antibodies on your sensitized mast cells. You'll recall that it is the binding of allergens and IgE antibodies that triggers an allergic reaction.

The extracts also cause your body to increase its production of suppressor T cells. These cells suppress the production of additional IgE antibodies. With fewer IgE antibodies in your system, you will be less likely to experience an allergic reaction.

Q: How much extract does each shot contain?

A: Initially, each injection contains a very small amount of the allergen protein in a special saltwater solution. Over a period of months, larger amounts of the protein are gradually added to the injection until the person reaches the maximum, or maintenance, dose of allergen.

Q: What about people who are allergic to more than one substance? Can the injection solution contain extracts of more than one allergen?

A: Yes. The solution can contain extracts of several allergens, all of which start at low concentrations, then gradually build up to the maintenance dose. People who are allergic to a large number of allergens may need several different injections at a time, each containing a different mix of allergen extracts. (Pollens are generally given together, while other allergens may be given in any number of combinations.) Multiple injections may also be given if a person is highly sensitive to a specific allergen. In such cases, the person receives that allergen separately, so it will not delay his desensitization to other allergens.

Q: Several injections at once! Do these injections hurt?

A: They are not comfortable, but they are not exceptionally painful. These injections, like those of the intradermal skin test, are given under the skin, not into the muscle, in alternating arms. And small needles are used.

Q: Who administers the shots?

A: The shots are generally administered by a doctor or nurse. Even if a nurse actually gives you the shots, a doctor is usually nearby to assist you in the event that you react to the shots.

Q: React in what way?

A: The most common side effect of allergy shots is swelling, redness or itching at the site of the injection. An oral antihistamine or aspirin usually relieves this minor discomfort. In other instances, the whole arm may swell. The most serious side effect, however, is anaphylaxis, which must be treated with a shot of epinephrine.

Fortunately, however, such extreme reactions are rare. And the risk of fatality from immunotherapy is rarer still (approximately one death per 2.5 million injections). Still, because the possibility of anaphylaxis exists, it is important that shots be administered only in a physician's office, where facilities and trained personnel are available to treat it. This is also why most doctors ask you to wait in the office for 20 to 30 minutes after you have received your shot. Most severe reactions to allergy shots occur during this time.

Q: How frequently are these injections given, and how long does it take to get to the maintenance dose?

A: Shots are typically administered once or twice a week to start. This schedule continues for approximately six months to a year until the maintenance dose is reached. At that point, the frequency decreases, gradually stretching to two, three or even four weeks.

Q: How is the maintenance dose determined?

A: The maintenance dose can be determined either by your doctor (typically a dose that researchers have found to be necessary for optimum relief) or by your own body. It's whichever comes first—the predetermined amount or the maximum dose you can tolerate without experiencing an allergic reaction.

Q: Are the shots given year-round?

A: Usually. Although allergy shots can be given seasonally— starting just before pollen season and continuing until the season is over, for example—most experts find that year-round immunotherapy is more effective.

Q: How long are the shots continued?

A: Immunotherapy is generally continued for three to five years, unless the patient fails to see improvement. If no improvement is seen within a year after a person reaches his maintenance dose, the shots are generally discontinued.

Q: I know people who have been getting allergy shots for a lot longer than five years. Why the discrepancy?

A: It is true that many doctors administer allergy shots indefinitely. But according to Harold Nelson, M.D., senior staff physician in the department of medicine at the National Jewish Center for Immunology and Respiratory Medicine in Denver, Colorado, "There seems to be little justification for most people in continuing for more than five years."

In the past, a lack of research, coupled with patients' fears of discontinuing the shots and doctors' willingness to continue administering the expensive treatments, made indefinite immunotherapy common. But Nelson predicts that will soon change.

Recent studies have proven that the effects of immunotherapy last after the shots are discontinued. Two studies—one involving grass pollen immunotherapy and one involving dust mite immunotherapy—found that the majority of people who undergo immunotherapy retain its benefits during the three years after they discontinued the shots. "The results are quite encouraging," Nelson says. "It doesn't appear that this should be a lifetime treatment."

Nelson believes that this research, along with the cost-consciousness of managed care, will likely lead to the development of practice parameters for immunotherapy. Once those parameters are set, "this endless immunotherapy will probably be diminishing."

Q: But immunotherapy will still require a long-term commitment, right?

A: Right. It takes some time—usually between six months and a year—before the effects of immunotherapy begin to be felt. And it takes still more time to achieve the maximum benefits of immunotherapy—generally at least three years. Some doctors advise continuing immunotherapy until a person has been symptom-free for two years.

If you are unable to commit to this long-term treatment, it may not be right for you.

Q: How will I know if immunotherapy is the right choice for me?

A: That's a decision you will have to make for yourself— after consulting with your doctor. Generally, the people who benefit most from immunotherapy are those who have a demonstrated allergy (confirmed by skin testing) to a substance for which allergen extracts are available; who experience allergy symptoms for at least several months of the year; who are unable to attain relief from those symptoms through medication or lifestyle changes; or who experience side effects from the medications used to treat their allergies.

Q: For what allergens are extracts available?

A: Extracts are available for pollens from a long list of trees, grasses and weeds as well as for dust mites, pet dander and indoor and outdoor molds—most of the common airborne allergens. Extracts for foods and other allergens are available as well; they are the same extracts used in skin testing. But because immunotherapy is generally not very effective for food allergies or allergies without respiratory symptoms, it is usually reserved for people who react to the common airborne allergens.

Q: I see. Are there any age limits for immunotherapy?

A: Immunotherapy is most successful in people ages 5 to 55. Treatment after age 55 is less effective, although it can provide relief for many people.

Q: If I were to decide to undergo immunotherapy, would I still need to take medication and alter my environment?

A: Yes. While your need for medication would probably decrease in time and perhaps disappear altogether, you would still need to avoid allergens as much as possible. As with other allergy treatments, avoidance is a key player in immunotherapy. It can greatly increase the effectiveness of the shots.

Q: What happens after the shots are discontinued?

A: That depends on the individual. As we said above, recent studies have shown that the majority of people continue to benefit from the shots even after they've been discontinued. Some people find that their sensitivity to allergens is permanently reduced. Others find that their symptoms return but are much less severe. But some find that their symptoms return in their original severity. There's no way to predict which people will experience this unfortunate circumstance, but these individuals do have the option of resuming immunotherapy.

Q: Didn't you say that immunotherapy is sometimes stopped early on because it doesn't result in improvement?

A: Yes. Although about 85 percent of people with allergic rhinitis obtain long-lasting relief with allergy shots, the remaining 15 percent do not. Unfortunately, there's no way of predicting who will and who will not respond to treatment.

Allergies to some substances do respond better than allergies to others, however.

Q: Which allergies respond best to immunotherapy?

A: The best results, as we've said, are seen in people who are allergic to airborne substances. Pollen allergies in general and ragweed allergy in particular usually respond well to immunotherapy, as do dust mite allergies. Allergies caused by molds do not respond as well. This is due in part to the quality of the extracts.

Q: What do you mean?

A: For allergy shots to work best, the extracts must contain an adequate amount of the specific substance to which the person is allergic. The methods for collecting extracts may vary, as may the amounts of allergens in the extracts. Some allergen extracts are purer than others. Pollen extracts, for example, are relatively pure; they are made from the allergenic pollen proteins. Mold extracts, on the other hand, are generally made from whole molds rather than from the allergenic spores. Extracts that are relatively pure, or those that have been standardized to contain a specific amount of allergen, are the most effective.

Q: What allergen extracts have been standardized?

A: Thus far, the Food and Drug Administration has standardized allergen extracts for cats, dust mites and ragweed; for the venoms of honeybees, yellow hornets, wasps, white-face hornets and yellow jackets; and for a mix of vespid venom. They are working on standardizing allergen extracts for a number of grass and tree pollens as well as for latex, cockroaches, peanuts and *Alternaria,* an indoor mold. Extracts for dogs, fire ants, seafood, dairy products, weed pollen allergens and the molds *Aspergillus* and *Hormodendrum* are slated for future standardization. In the meantime, nonstandardized extracts of these and other allergens are available. These extracts may not be as effective as their standardized counterparts, but they should provide some relief.

Q: **With the exception of the insect venoms, most of the allergens in that list are airborne. I know you said allergy shots are generally used to manage allergic rhinitis, but are they effective in treating any other allergies?**

A: Yes. As you may assume from the above list, insect venom immunotherapy can be very successful, often providing complete protection against future stings. And on certain occasions—generally when a person is in urgent need of a drug for which there is no substitute—an accelerated version of immunotherapy can be used to treat drug allergy. You'll recall that we discussed both of these types of immunotherapy in chapter 6.

Q: **What about asthma? Didn't you say that immunotherapy is used to treat asthma?**

A: Immunotherapy is used to treat some people with asthma.

Q: **Some people? Which ones?**

A: Immunotherapy can help about half of the 40 to 60 percent of asthmatic people with allergies—people who meet three criteria.

Q: **And those criteria are . . . ?**

A: (1) The person must have allergic asthma caused by one specific allergy; (2) the person must have first tried to control his asthma with allergen avoidance and drug therapy but found the control insufficient; and (3) the person should have at least some control over his asthma.

Q: If immunotherapy is a success, does it cure asthma?

A: There is as yet no cure for asthma. But if allergy shots work well, they can reduce or eliminate the reaction to certain triggers as well as reduce the amount of medication needed to control the disease.

In one study, asthmatic people with ragweed allergies who underwent two years of immunotherapy had higher peak-flow readings and fewer emergency room visits than those who did not undergo allergy shots. The people on immunotherapy needed less than half of the asthma medication of those who didn't undergo allergy shots—leading doctors to postulate that the cost of immunotherapy could be offset, in part, by lower medication costs.

Q: That reminds me. Didn't you say allergy shots are expensive?

A: Yes. Although prices vary nationwide, a five-year course of immunotherapy may cost in excess of $5,000. Fortunately, most types of insurance cover at least part of the bill.

Q: I bet a lot of that goes to pay the doctor's or nurse's salary. Couldn't I give myself my own allergy shots?

A: In some instances—most notably in isolated areas where doctors are few and far between—allergy patients do indeed administer their own allergy shots. This is a matter of controversy among allergists. The major concern, as we've just seen, is the possibility that the person may experience a life-threatening anaphylactic reaction at home, where appropriate medical care is unavailable. The American Academy of Allergy, Asthma and Immunology has issued position statements against home administration of allergy shots, noting the risks it poses for the patient, including possible complications from errors in administration, underestimation of symptoms, unawareness of the early symptoms of anaphylaxis and the inability to administer lifesaving therapy.

In short, it is always preferable to receive the shots in a doctor's office. But in cases where that is not possible, some doctors instruct patients how to administer the shots, let them know what side effects they should be concerned about and teach them how to use injectable epinephrine in the event that a systemic reaction occurs.

Q: **I know you said these reactions are rare, but is there any chance the safety of immunotherapy will be improved in the future? The benefits appeal to me, but going to the doctor's office and sitting there for 20 minutes every few weeks isn't my idea of fun.**

A: The safety as well as the efficacy of immunotherapy is being improved with the advent of increasingly potent, standardized allergen extracts. Researchers are also working to improve the way the extracts are delivered.

An experimental form of nasal immunotherapy that has few, if any, side effects is now being tested. In a 1995 study, Italian researchers found that patients allergic to *Parietaria* pollen, a common Mediterranean allergen, showed substantial improvement in allergy symptoms when they were given twice a week, increasing doses of pollen in dried form by nasal inhaler in the six months prior to the allergy season. Because the nasal immunotherapy produced no side effects, researchers speculate that it may be safe enough for patients to administer on their own.

Research is also underway to develop an oral immunotherapy in which people with allergies could receive their extracts in capsule form. Oral immunotherapy has proven less effective than standard immunotherapy in the past, primarily because it requires much larger doses of extract and more time to achieve the maintenance dose. But a new technique for encapsulating allergen extract may make oral immunotherapy an option, according to researchers at the University of Cincinnati College of Medicine. In the researchers' 1996 study, patients given gelatin capsules containing ragweed extract achieved a therapeutic dose in seven weeks and experienced no side effects.

Meanwhile, researchers at Johns Hopkins University are experimenting with injections that contain peptide fragments—pieces of proteins—of the allergens instead of whole-allergen extracts. This "vaccine" form of immunotherapy appears to lower the risk of severe reaction.

Until these strategies are perfected, however, standard immunotherapy—involving periodic allergy shots—remains the only way to actually alter a person's sensitivity to an allergen.

INFORMATIONAL AND MUTUAL-AID GROUPS

Allergy and Asthma Network/Mothers of Asthmatics, Inc.
3554 Chain Bridge Rd., Suite 200, Fairfax, VA 22030
800-878-4403

Provides patient education and information on asthma and allergies; sells publications and videos. Individual membership ($25) includes a subscription to the MA Report, *a monthly newsletter.*

American Academy of Allergy, Asthma and Immunology
611 E. Wells St., Milwaukee, WI 53202
414-272-6071
800-822-2762
http://www.aaaai.org

Professional organization for allergists; provides information on asthma and allergies and offers regional listings of allergy specialists; publishes the Journal of Allergy and Clinical Immunology.

American College of Allergy, Asthma and Immunology
85 W. Algonquin, Suite 550, Arlington Heights, IL 60005
312-359-2800
800-842-7777
http://allergy.mcg.edu

Professional association for allergists; provides information on allergies and asthma and offers state listings of physicians specializing in allergy; publishes the Annals of Allergy, Asthma and Immunology.

Asthma and Allergy Foundation of America
1125 15th St. NW, Suite 502, Washington, DC 20005
202-466-7643
800-7ASTHMA (727-8462)

Supports research on asthma and allergies; offers patient education programs; sells publications. Individual membership ($25) includes a subscription to the bimonthly newsletter Advance *and a discount on publications.*

163

The Food Allergy Network
10400 Eaton Pl., Suite 107, Fairfax, VA 22030-2208
703-691-3179
800-929-4040
http://www.foodallergy.org

Works to increase public awareness about food allergies; offers publications and videos. Individual membership ($24) includes a subscription to the bimonthly newsletter Food Allergy News *and consumer alerts.*

National Heart, Lung and Blood Institute
National Asthma Education Program
P.O. Box 30105, Bethesda, MD 20824-0103
301-251-1222

Provides information on asthma to patients and professionals.

National Institute of Allergy and Infectious Diseases
Office of Communications
9000 Rockville Pike, Bethesda, MD 20892
301-496-5717
http://www.niaid.nih.gov

Conducts and supports research on infectious and allergic diseases; offers publications.

National Jewish Center for Immunology and Respiratory Medicine
1400 Jackson St., Denver, CO 80206
303-398-1079
800-222-LUNG

Provides information on allergies, asthma and other respiratory diseases.

GLOSSARY

Albumin: Allergenic protein found in egg whites.

Allergens: Normally harmless foreign substances that cause an allergic response.

Allergic asthma: See **Extrinsic asthma**.

Allergic conjunctivitis: Inflammation of the membrane lining of the eye (conjunctiva) caused by allergy.

Allergic contact dermatitis: Skin rash resulting from contact with an allergenic substance.

Allergic rhinitis: Inflammation of the nasal passages caused by allergy; often accompanied by nasal discharge and itching of the nose and eyes.

Allergic rhinoconjunctivitis: Inflammation of the nasal passages and eyes caused by allergy.

Allergic salute: Characteristic rubbing of the nose to relieve nasal itching; often leaves a crease on the bridge of the nose.

Allergic shiner: Swelling of the blood vessels under the eye caused by allergy.

Allergist: Physician who specializes in diagnosing and treating allergy.

Allergy: Abnormal immune system reaction to a generally harmless substance.

Allergy shots: See **Immunotherapy**.

Anaphylactic shock: Severe and sometimes fatal allergic response to an allergen characterized by low blood pressure and breathing difficulties.

Anaphylactoid reaction: Severe response to a foreign substance that is not triggered by the immune system (i.e., not allergic in nature).

Anaphylaxis: The most severe type of allergic reaction; a severe and sometimes fatal systemic allergic reaction that may include swelling, hives, low blood pressure, breathing difficulties and, in some instances, shock and heart failure.

Angioedema: Swelling of deep skin tissue common to the face, neck, lips, throat, hands, feet, genitals and abdominal organs; often caused by allergy.

Antibodies: Substances made by the immune system to neutralize antigens or allergens.

Antigens: Substances foreign to the body that cause the immune system to form antibodies.

Antihistamine: A drug that counteracts histamine in the body; used to treat allergic reactions and colds.

Apids: Stinging insects of the Hymenoptera class; honeybees.

Applied kinesiology: Controversial allergy test that measures changes in a patient's muscle strength before and after he is exposed to an allergen.

Aquagenic urticaria: Hives caused by contact with water.

Asthma: Inflammatory disease in which air passages of the lungs periodically become narrowed, obstructed or blocked. Typical symptoms include shortness of breath, wheezing, chest tightness and coughing.

Atopic: Adjective describing the hereditary tendency to develop immediate allergic reactions such as asthma, eczema and allergic rhinitis.

Atopic dermatitis: Itchy skin rash commonly found on the face, knees and elbows of allergy-prone people. Also called eczema.

Basophils: White blood cells that circulate through the bloodstream and release histamine during allergic reactions.

B cells: See **B lymphocytes**.

B lymphocytes: White blood cells responsible for humoral immunity; B lymphocytes trigger the creation of antibodies.

Body chemical analysis: Controversial allergy test that measures various chemicals in body fluids and tissues in an attempt to diagnose allergy.

Bronchioles: Small airways from the bronchi to the lobes of the lungs that allow the exchange of air and waste gases.

Bronchodilators: Drugs that relax airway muscles, thus opening the airways.

Bronchospasms: Tiny muscle spasms or constrictions in the muscles that encircle the bronchial air passages, resulting in airway narrowing; a symptom of asthma.

Casein: Allergenic protein in milk.

Cell-mediated immunity: Type of immunity granted by T lymphocytes that helps the body resist infection and is responsible for delayed allergic responses.

Cholinergic urticaria: Hives caused by an increase in the body's core temperature; this increase can be caused either by direct exposure to heat or hot water or by exercise and anxiety.

Chronic obstructive pulmonary disease (COPD): Incurable condition in which lungs are able to take in less air over a period of time, resulting in breathing difficulties.

Cleft palate: Birth defect in which there is a hole in the middle of the roof of the mouth.

Clinical ecology: Alternative approach to medicine that ascribes a wide range of symptoms to exposure to common substances in the environment; clinical ecology theory holds that these sensitivities, sometimes referred to as allergies, are related to a malfunction of the immune system; also called environmental medicine.

Cold urticaria: Hives caused by exposure to cold.

Conjunctiva: The membrane that lines the inner surface of the eyelid and the front part of the white of the eye.

Contact dermatitis: Skin rash caused by contact with an allergen or irritant.

COPD: See **Chronic obstructive pulmonary disease**.

Corticosteroids: Drugs that prevent or reduce inflammation; used to treat a variety of allergic conditions.

Cromolyn sodium: Anti-inflammatory drug that stabilizes mast cells.

Cross-reactivity: Allergic reaction to a substance caused by allergy to a similar substance.

Cytotoxic test: Controversial allergy test that looks for changes in a person's white blood cells after a sample of his blood is placed on a microscope slide that has been smeared with dried food extract.

Dander: Sloughed-off skin flakes; animal dander can be highly allergenic.

Decongestants: Drugs used to reduce congestion or swelling, especially in the nasal passages.

Delayed hypersensitivity: Allergic reaction that occurs some time after exposure to an allergen; a form of cell-mediated immune response.

Dermatographism: Abnormal skin condition in which large raised areas result when a blunt object is drawn across the skin.

Desensitization: Process by which a person sensitive to various allergens is made insensitive to those allergens. See also **Immunotherapy**.

Deviated septum: Condition in which the center section of the nose shifts to one side.

Diuretics: Drugs that promote urination, thus speeding the body's elimination of sodium and water; often used to control blood pressure.

Dust mites: Microscopic arachnids that live in dust, carpeting and upholstery; their feces and body parts are highly allergenic.

Eczema: See **Atopic dermatitis**.

Electrodermal diagnosis: Controversial allergy test that measures changes in the electrical resistance of a person's skin when he is exposed to an allergen.

Environmental medicine: See **Clinical ecology**.

Eosinophils: White blood cells that are present in large numbers with allergy.

Epinephrine: Hormonelike drug that stimulates the adrenal glands and narrows blood vessels; used to treat anaphylaxis.

Erythema: Redness and swelling of the skin.

Eustachian tubes: Tubes that connect the ears to the nose-throat cavity; can become blocked by allergy, causing ear infection and hearing loss.

Exercise-induced anaphylaxis: Anaphylaxis that is triggered by exercise; usually occurs when a person eats before exercising.

Extrinsic asthma: Form of asthma triggered by allergy.

Food diary: Written record of all foods eaten during a specified time period; used to diagnose food allergy.

Food elimination and challenge tests: Tests in which specific foods are eliminated from the diet or introduced to the diet; used to diagnose food allergy.

H_1 antihistamines: Antihistamines that compete with histamine to connect with H_1 receptors; the mainstays of allergy treatment.

H_2 antihistamines: Antihistamines that compete with histamine to connect with H_2 receptors; occasionally used in conjunction with H_1 antihistamines to treat chronic hives.

Hay fever: See **Seasonal allergic rhinitis**.

Histamine: Chemical mediator released in allergic reactions that widens blood vessels, lowers blood pressure, releases gastric juices, contracts smooth muscles and irritates nerve endings.

Histamine-releasing factor (HRF): Protein that, when combined with a certain antibody, appears to affect the severity and duration of allergic reactions.

Hives: See **Urticaria**.

HRF: See **Histamine-releasing factor**.

Humoral immunity: Form of immunity provided by the development and presence of antibodies.

Hymenoptera: Class of stinging insects that includes vespids and apids.

Idiopathic: Of unknown cause.

IgE: Immunoglobulin E; class of immunoglobulins that is responsible for allergic reactions.

IgG: Immunoglobulin G; class of immunoglobulins that responds to bacteria, fungi and viruses; increases during immunotherapy.

Immune system: Complex system that protects the body from disease organisms and other foreign bodies; includes the humoral immune response and the cell-mediated immune response.

Immunoglobulin: Any of five classes of antibodies in bodily fluids.

Immunology: Study of the reaction of tissues of the immune system to stimulation by antigens.

Immunotherapy: Desensitizing treatment for allergy; involves injections of increasingly large doses of offending allergens in an effort to build up immunity to those allergens.

Inhalant allergens: Allergens that are inhaled or airborne.

Intolerance: Nonallergic adverse reaction to a substance such as a food or drug.

Intracutaneous test: See **Intradermal test**.

Intradermal test: Allergy skin test in which extracts of allergens are injected into the skin; the skin is observed to determine if it reacts to the allergens.

In vitro histamine release: Test that detects the release of histamine from basophils in blood exposed to an allergen in a test tube; used for research purposes.

In vitro lymphocyte proliferation: Blood test that gives a picture of cell-mediated immunity.

Ipratropium bromide: An anticholinergic drug used to open the airways in people with asthma; also used to stop runny nose in people with allergic rhinitis.

Irritants: Substances that irritate the body.

Lactose: Sugar found in milk.

Leukocytes: White blood cells.

Leukotriene receptor antagonists: Asthma drugs that compete with leukotrienes to reach leukotriene receptors.

Leukotrienes: Chemical compounds in the body that occur in white blood cells and are able to produce allergic and inflammatory reactions; mediators.

Lichenification: Thickening and hardening of the skin that's often the result of irritation caused by repeated scratching of an itchy rash.

Lymph: Thin, clear fluid that circulates through the lymphatic system.

Lymphatic system: System of vessels, nodes and organs that produces, filters and conveys lymph and produces various blood cells.

Lymphocytes: Small white blood cells that play an important role in the immune system; there are two types—B lymphocytes, or B cells, and T lymphocytes, or T cells.

Lymphokines: Chemicals produced and released by T lymphocytes that attract phagocytes to the site of an infection or inflammation.

Mast cells: Cells in connective tissue that contain histamine and other substances.

Mast-cell stabilizers: Drugs that stabilize mast cells, preventing them from releasing antihistamine and other mediators.

Mediators: Chemicals that mediate, or act on, various components of the immune system; these chemicals provoke inflammation and cause the symptoms of allergic reactions.

Mold counts: Counts that identify the number of mold spores per cubic meter of outdoor air.

Molds: Simple plants in the fungus family; molds reproduce by spores, which are highly allergenic.

Mucokinetic drugs: Drugs that help clear mucus from the lungs.

Mucosa: Mucous membrane; a thin sheet of tissue cells that cover or line various parts of the body.

Multiple chemical sensitivity: Controversial condition in which a person is sensitive to numerous substances in the environment.

Nasal polyps: Long, round bits of overgrown mucous membrane that extend into the nasal cavity.

Neutrophils: Circulating white blood cells that remove and destroy bacteria, cell debris and solid particles in the blood.

Nonsteroidal anti-inflammatory drugs (NSAIDs): Drugs that do not contain steroids used to reduce inflammation.

NSAIDs: See **Nonsteroidal anti-inflammatory drugs**.

Occupational allergic rhinitis: Allergic rhinitis triggered by allergens a person is exposed to at work.

Ocular: Pertaining to the eye.

Oral allergy syndrome: Itching and swelling of the lips and tongue after eating a food to which one is allergic.

Ovalbumin: Allergenic protein in egg whites.

Patch test: Allergy skin test in which an allergen is applied directly to the skin for a certain period of time; used to diagnose delayed hypersensitivity allergies such as allergic contact dermatitis.

Perennial allergic rhinitis: Form of allergic rhinitis that occurs year-round; often caused by indoor allergens such as mold, dust, dust mites and animal dander.

Phagocytes: Immune system cells that engulf and digest organisms and cell waste.

Photoallergic reactions: Allergic reactions after exposure to light.

Placebo: An inactive substance.

Pollen counts: Number of pollen grains per cubic meter of outdoor air.

Pollens: Fertilizing elements of flowering plants; fine, powdery yellow grains.

Postnasal drip: Drop-by-drop release of nasal mucus into the back of the throat; a symptom of nasal allergy.

Pressure urticaria: Hives caused by pressure applied to the skin.

Prick test: Allergy skin test in which allergen extracts are placed on the skin, then the skin is pricked and observed for allergic reactions.

Prophylactic: Preventive.

Prostaglandins: Hormonelike fatty acids that act on certain organs; in allergy, they act as chemical mediators.

Provocation-neutralization: Controversial allergy test in which a patient is given varying concentrations of extracts of suspected allergens either by injection or sublingually. Any sensations or symptoms, which indicate a positive reaction, are then neutralized with a dose of the same substance.

Pruritus: Itching.

Pseudoallergic reactions: Reactions that are not caused by allergy but that resemble allergic reactions.

Pulmonary function tests: Tests that determine how well the lungs are performing and estimate the severity of airway obstruction.

Puncture test: See **Prick test.**

Radioallergosorbent test (RAST): Blood test that measures the amount of specific IgE antibodies in the blood; used to diagnose or confirm specific allergies.

Radiocontrast media: Radioactive dyes used in x-ray, computerized axial tomography (CAT) scans and other tests to help the radiologist see the organs being studied.

Radioimmunosorbent test (RIST): Blood test that measures the total amount of IgE antibodies in the blood; used to determine if a person has allergies.

Ragweed: Woody herb with a highly allergenic pollen.

RAST: See **Radioallergosorbent test.**

Reaginic pulse test: Controversial allergy test in which a person's pulse is measured before and after he is exposed to an allergen.

Receptors: Areas of nerve endings and certain cells that respond to specific kinds of action.

Rhinitis medicamentosa: Form of nasal inflammation caused by medication—generally topical decongestants.

Rhinorrhea: Runny nose.

Rhinoscope: Magnifying device used to examine the nasal passages.

RIST: See **Radioimmunosorbent test**.

Rose fever: Term for seasonal allergic rhinitis that occurs in the spring.

Scratch test: Allergy skin test in which allergy extracts are placed on a lightly scratched area of skin, then observed to see if an allergic reaction occurs.

Seasonal allergic rhinitis: Allergic rhinitis that occurs only during certain times of the year; usually caused by seasonal allergens such as pollens and mold spores.

Sensitization: An acquired reaction in which specific antibodies develop in response to an antigen, or allergen.

Sick building syndrome: Situation in which people experience a variety of symptoms in reaction to allergens and irritants in an indoor environment without adequate ventilation.

Sinusitis: Inflammation of the nasal sinuses; a complication of allergy.

Solar urticaria: Hives caused by exposure to sunlight or, occasionally, artificial light.

Spores: Reproductive bodies of certain simple organisms; molds reproduce by spores.

Sulfa drugs: See **Sulfonamides**.

Sulfites: Preservatives used in processed foods and beverages—including processed shellfish and mushrooms, potato chips, dried fruits and wine—that trigger allergy-like reactions such as rhinitis, hives, asthma flare-ups and anaphylaxis.

Sulfonamides: Allergenic group of drugs used to treat infections; also called sulfa drugs.

Tartrazine: An allergenic yellow food dye.

T cells: See **T lymphocytes**.

Thymus: A gland that is part of the immune system; where T lymphocytes mature.

T lymphocytes: White blood cells responsible for cell-mediated immunity.

Urticaria: Skin eruption caused by histamine and other mediators and marked by transient wheals of varying shapes and sizes with clear margins and pale centers; often an allergic reaction to foods, drugs or insect bites or stings; also called hives.

Urushiol: Highly allergenic oily resin found on poison ivy, poison oak and poison sumac.

Vespids: Stinging insects of the Hymenoptera class; yellow jackets, hornets and wasps.

Wheal: A patch of itchy skin, often raised.

Wheezing: Whistling or rasping sound heard during inhalation or exhalation caused by airflow through narrowed airways; a symptom of asthma.

Whey: Proteins in milk.

SUGGESTED READING

American Academy of Allergy, Asthma and Immunology. "Adverse Reactions to Foods." Pamphlet. August 1993.

American Academy of Allergy, Asthma and Immunology. "What Every Patient Should Know About Asthma and Allergy." Pamphlet. November 1992.

Anderson, John A., M.D. "Allergic Reactions to Drugs and Biological Agents." *Journal of the American Medical Association* 268 (November 25, 1992): 2845-2857.

Bernstein, Leonard I., M.D., and William W. Storms, M.D. "Practice Parameters for Allergy Diagnostic Testing." *Annals of Allergy, Asthma & Immunology* 75 (December 1995): 543-625.

Boggs, Peter B., M.D. *Sneezing Your Head Off? How to Live With Your Allergic Nose.* New York: Fireside, 1992.

Claman, Henry N., M.D. "The Biology of the Immune Response." *Journal of the American Medical Association* 268 (November 25, 1992): 2790-2796.

Creticos, Peter S., M.D. "Immunotherapy With Allergens." *Journal of the American Medical Association* 268 (November 25, 1992): 2834-2839.

Horan, Richard F., M.D., Lynda C. Schneider, M.D., and Albert Sheffer, M.D. "Allergic Skin Disorders and Mastocytosis." *Journal of the American Medical Association* 268 (November 25, 1992): 2858-2868.

Isselbacher, Kurt J., A.B., M.D., Eugene Braunwald, A.B., M.D., Jean D. Wilson, M.D., Joseph B. Martin, M.D., Ph.D., FRCP, Anthony S. Fauci, M.D., Dennis L. Kasper, M.D., editors. *Harrison's Principles of Internal Medicine.* 13th ed. New York: McGraw-Hill Inc., 1994.

Joneja, Janice M. Vickerstaff, Ph.D., and Leonard Bielory, M.D. *Understanding Allergy, Sensitivity and Immunity: A Comprehensive Guide.* New Brunswick, N.J.: Rutgers University Press, 1990.

Kaliner, Michael, M.D., and Robert Lemanske, M.D. "Rhinitis and Asthma." *Journal of the American Medical Association* 268 (November 25, 1992): 2807-2829.

Reisman, Robert E., M.D. "Insect Stings." *New England Journal of Medicine* 331 (August 25, 1994): 523-527.

Sampson, Hugh A., M.D., and Dean D. Metcalfe, M.D. "Food Allergies." *Journal of the American Medical Association* 268 (November 25, 1992): 2840-2844.

Schultz, Nathan D., M.D., Allan V. Giannini, M.D., Terrance T. Chang, M.D., and Diane C. Wong. *The Best Guide to Allergy.* 3d ed. Totowa, N.J.: Humana Press, 1994.

Simmons, F. Estelle R., M.D., and Keith J. Simons, Ph.D. "The Pharmacology and Use of H_1 Receptor Antagonist Drugs." *New England Journal of Medicine* 330 (June 9, 1994): 1663-1669.

Valentine, Martin D., M.D. "Anaphylaxis and Stinging Insect Hypersensitivity." *Journal of the American Medical Association* 268 (November 25, 1992): 2830-2833.

Weinstein, Allan M., M.D. *Asthma: The Complete Guide to Self-Management of Asthma and Allergies for Patients and Their Families.* New York: Ballantine, 1988.

Young, Stuart H., M.D., Bruce S. Dobozin, M.D., Margaret Miner and the editors of Consumer Reports Books. *Allergies: The Complete Guide to Diagnosis, Treatment and Daily Management.* Yonkers, N.Y.: Consumer Reports Books, 1991.

ON-LINE RESOURCES

The following Web sites provide information about allergies and asthma.

http://www.allerdays.com

Provides information on allergies, pollen seasons and research.

http://www.allergy-info.com

Provides information on allergy management, local pollen and mold spore counts and allergy medications; sponsored by Pfizer Inc. and UCB Pharma.

http://www.allergyrelief.com

Provides information on seasonal rhinitis and allergy medications; sponsored by Schering-Plough.

http://www.allergyshop.com

Provides general information about allergies; sponsored by The Allergy Shop.

http://www.eznet.net/aarrc

Provides information on allergies; sponsored by Allergy and Asthma Rochester Resource Center, Ltd.

http://www.niaid.nih.gov

Provides information on allergies; sponsored by the National Institute of Allergy and Infectious disease.

http://www.sig.net/~allergy

Provides general information about allergies; sponsored by Allergy Center.

http://www.foodallergy.org

Provides information about food allergies; sponsored by the Food Allergy Network.

http://www.aaaai.org

Provides information on allergies and asthma; sponsored by the American Academy of Allergy, Asthma and Immunology.

http://allergy.mcg.edu

Provides information on allergies and asthma; sponsored by the American College of Allergy, Asthma and Immunology.

INDEX